PRAISE FOR MALE 2.0

"As a thought leader in men's health, Dr. Gapin has provided the modern-day blueprint to help men optimize their health and regain their vitality. Every man should read this book."

JJ Virgin

NYT Bestselling Author of *The Virgin Diet & Sugar Impact Diet* as featured on Dr. Phil, Dr. Oz, and the Today Show

"Dr. Gapin saved my sexual life and this book continues to improve my lifestyle. My genetic test result was like reading a horoscope except it was accurate. It changed the way I approached life."

Paul Nolting

Learning Specialist

"I was seeking a major change. I was tired of being pitched boilerplate diet and exercise strategies. I wanted a customized solution for me. The Male 2.0 approach delivered a finely tuned regimen of diet, exercise, supplements and peptides. Results? I lost 30 pounds, don't ache every morning, and I sleep better! Feel better and live longer with Male 2.0!"

Andrew Cardone

Wealth Advisor Executive

MALE 2.0

TRACY BRIAN GAPIN, MD, FACS

MALE 2.0

CRACKING THE CODE TO LIMITLESS HEALTH AND VITALITY

TRACY BRIAN GAPIN, MD, FACS

MALE 2.0

Cracking the Code to Limitless Health and Vitality

Gapin Institute, LLC
5911 N. Honore Ave #103
Sarasota, FL 34243

ISBN: 978-0-578-60596-8

Cover Design by Ash Ahern

Interior Design by Transcendent Publishing

Disclaimer: This book is not intended to diagnose, treat, cure, or prevent any disease and is not intended to be the medical advice of a physician. The reader should regularly consult a physician in matters relating to his/her health and particularly with respect to any symptoms that may require diagnosis or medical attention.

Printed in the United States of America.

DEDICATION

To my amazing children, Graham and Reese, and my beautiful wife, Sara, who inspire me to be a better father, husband and man.

And to all the men striving to be the best version of themselves for the people they love.

CONTENTS

PREFACE

finished writing this book in early 2020. It was ready for publication when everything changed. The coronavirus pandemic exploded and profoundly changed our lives forever.

Hundreds of thousands of people lost their lives. Millions suffered with significant health-related symptoms. And nearly everyone felt the catastrophic economic impact.

So, what did we learn from it all? What can we take away from this life-altering event? Is there a silver lining to be found? Some statistics about the mortality from COVID-19 can refine our perspective.

A recent JAMA study evaluated the health characteristics of 5700 patients hospitalized in New York due to the coronavirus[2]. They found that the mortality rate in men was much higher than in women. And they found older age was associated with increased mortality.

But the critical information from this study centered around chronic health issues such as hypertension (high blood pressure), obesity, diabetes, and cardiovascular disease. These health issues were found to be associated with worse outcomes from COVID-19.

In patients who required hospitalization, only 6% had no chronic health issues, whereas 88% of them had at least two. And only 2.1% of those who died were healthy with no such comorbidities.

So, what's the take-home message here?

It's time to take control of your health. If you wait until you get sick, it's too late. It's time to start optimizing your health NOW.

It's time to be proactive and invest in your future.

It's time for MALE 2.0.

INTRODUCTION

I had never felt quite so vulnerable. There I sat on the exam table, wearing only a thin gown that didn't do much to cover me. It was a scene I knew well — a doctor's office, exam table, and sterile-looking cabinets all around. I'd spent almost every day for nearly twenty years in a room just like this one. But this time it was different, because this time I was the patient.

What in the world was I doing here? I had never been to see a doctor before. I'd always been healthy, so why would I?

But I knew something was very wrong with me. I was stressed out, I felt like crap, and I wasn't sleeping well. I had also lost interest in sex. Seriously? A guy my age, not interested in sex?! I didn't really know what rock bottom was, but I felt like I was close.

I had spent years taking care of my family, tending to my patients, and building a career I had been working towards since I was a kid. And, like so many busy men, I had neglected my own health in the process. I was working crazy hours, living on junk food, not exercising, and generally treating my body like trash.

I was so focused on taking care of everyone else I had lost sight of my own health. More importantly, I was failing those who I cared about more than anything — my wife and kids.

That's how at age forty-two, I found myself in that doctor's office for my very first physical exam ever. And the news wasn't good. I was thirty pounds overweight, had high cholesterol, diminished kidney function, and signs of chronic inflammation. I wasn't exactly "sick", but I was far from healthy. I was also, for the first time in my life, aware of my own mortality, and it was scary.

More shocking than the test results was my new doctor's advice.

"Tracy, you just need to drink more water, eat more vegetables and exercise more. And maybe take a statin." That was it.

I left his office not just scared but a little confused. I had gone to him looking for answers and water, vegetables, exercise and "maybe a statin" didn't seem to cut it.

Worse still was the realization that as a doctor, I didn't know any more than he did. In fact, some of my own patients had come to me with similar problems. But despite four years of medical school, six years of surgical residency, and years of practice as a surgeon saving lives every day, I didn't have any better answers.

Before I go any further, let me introduce myself. My name is Dr. Tracy Gapin — "Doc Tracy" to my patients. I'm a board-certified urologist, a men's health expert, and a bit of a rebel.

For almost twenty years guys just like me had come into my office, and I hadn't been able to help them get healthy, just like my doctor couldn't help me. Why? Because medical school and residency training do not teach us how to truly get to the root of these issues and resolve them. We learn how to treat symptoms and how to treat disease, but not how to actually help our patients be healthy.

Clearly, something had to change. That was the beginning of my quest to find a better way, and the result of that quest was Male 2.0™.

CHAPTER ONE

MALE 1.0

Before getting to the solution, let me first delve a little bit deeper into the problem. It's a problem that affects all men, regardless of age.

We are experiencing a men's health crisis, a full-blown epidemic that nobody wants to talk about. If you're a guy, you are either already affected by it, or it's only a matter of time before you will be.

It all starts with a T for Testosterone. As you will see, it doesn't end there. But it definitely starts there.

Here's a frightening fact: testosterone levels are plummeting. They have dropped more than 30% over the last thirty years, and if things don't change, it's only going to get worse.

At the current rate, in twenty years the entire male population will be sterile and impotent.

Maybe you're thinking, why should I care? I've already had my kids and in twenty years I'll be too old to care about sex. Here's the thing — testosterone is not just about procreation or sexual activity, it's what makes you a man. As we will discuss a little later, testosterone is also critical for normal energy level, cognitive function, and athletic performance. You need healthy testosterone levels to build muscle and burn fat. You need it to maintain healthy bone density and a healthy cardiovascular system. In fact, some have suggested that low testosterone may be the *underlying cause* of cardiovascular disease. Think about the massive implications of that!

Low testosterone for guys in their forties, fifties and sixties is catastrophic. It's the reason midlife leads to weight gain, poor sleep, deteriorating physical and cognitive performance, and diminished sexual function.

Maybe you feel like you've lost your edge. Maybe you don't know what the hell happened to the virile, happy, strong, energetic guy you used to be and are wondering how to find him again. Or maybe you've given up, figuring your best years are behind you and that this is your new reality.

Maybe, if you're like the guys I see in my office every day, you have no idea what to do about it, so you take the path of least resistance and do nothing... nothing until you've reached rock bottom and your life is a total mess.

Where'd You Go, Joe?

Joe sat in my office, looking at me helplessly through the eyes of a tired old man. He was hoping I'd give him a testosterone shot and send him on his way. Joe may have been impatient, but he didn't have much fighting spirit.

He had been happily married with two kids and a great job, but over the past five to ten years, everything had changed. He had become incredibly fatigued, depressed and uninterested in life. Joe struggled just to get through each day, often by drowning himself in cup after cup of coffee. Eventually it affected his performance as a C-suite executive, and he lost his job.

He had gained about twenty pounds of weight from his baseline, and he had no desire to do anything about it. He was too tired to go to a gym, and even if he could summon the energy, he didn't really know what he would do when he got there.

It affected his relationship with his family as well. He no longer had interest in playing sports with his kids, and he had absolutely no interest in sex. And forget about sexual function. His wife actually started to suspect that he was having an affair, which led to other problems between them and eventually the demise of their sixteen-year-marriage.

Joe told me how his entire personality and mood had changed. He'd somehow gone from strong, happy and eager to depressed, frustrated, and tired. As he sat before me in the office, I was struck by how defeated he looked.

What had happened to Joe to cause such a dramatic change in his life? Well, nothing and everything. Nothing, because it wasn't any single, unexpected event; everything because so many things had happened to Joe all at once. And, over the course of the previous ten years, they had caused him to stop being the man he used to be.

"How did I get so old, Doctor?" Joe asked me pointedly.

Joe wasn't old at all. He was barely in his forties. But when I ran his labs, his testosterone levels were on par with a man *in his eighties*.

Though Joe was a new patient, I felt like I had met him a hundred times before, and in a way I had. Guys like him walked into my office every day, and over the course of my two decades as a doctor, they had gotten younger and younger. Sometimes, they were still in their twenties and looked just as exhausted and defeated as Joe.

I've seen so many guys settle for living this way and miss out on a lot of years of quality living, solely because they have no idea that there's a problem that can be resolved. At that point, my first order of business is to convince guys to want to pick up the pieces and get back to life as they knew it.

A guy dealing with low testosterone may not be facing a life or death situation… yet. But my focus goes well beyond saving lives, or even improving them. It's about *optimizing* lives. It's about optimizing health and performance so that men of any age can enjoy life without limitations and be the best version of themselves. So they can be limitless.

Don't Be Late to the Party, Marty

Marty came into my office one day, and just like Joe, he was eager to get a testosterone shot. He had a stoicism about him that Joe didn't have, despite being morbidly obese.

Marty exhibited a surprising lack of concern about his weight or any other aspect of his health. He just wanted his youthful libido and bedroom performance back. Actually "want" is an over-statement; he had only come to see me, he admitted, because his wife's nagging had become so unbearable.

When I expressed concern about his weight and overall health, he replied impatiently, "What does it matter, Doc? My dad was fat and diabetic, and so is my sister. It's only a matter of time before I am too. Can you just give me a testosterone shot?"

Marty knew he had a problem, one he thought could be fixed with a simple injection. It never occurred to him that his poor libido and sexual function, weight, and overall health were all tied to-gether.

You know what else he didn't consider? That despite his family history, he could lose weight, get back the energy he had years ago, get healthy and avoid diabetes. His genetics didn't dictate his destiny. More to come on that later!

I couldn't really blame Marty, because his approach to his health was the classic case of Male 1.0. What do I mean by that? He was operating from the same system I was taught in medical school and residency, namely, the disease model. The one where you wait until you're "sick" to go see a doctor, who then focuses on treating or managing your symptoms until the next time you're "sick." In the meantime, you just trudge through life.

Marty was just doing what was expected of him, and he was expecting exactly what our disease model system is set up for: take some medication or treatment that masks symptoms but never deals with the underlying issues.

As I mentioned earlier, the problem begins with testosterone, but it doesn't end there. I know, because I see it every day. Men are also dealing with obesity, cardiovascular disease, elevated cholesterol levels, insulin resistance (an early form of diabetes), and depression. There is an increasing incidence of what's called "metabolic syndrome." This is a constellation of at least three of the following: central obesity (belly fat), high blood pressure, elevated blood sugar, high triglycerides, and low HDL cholesterol. Metabolic syndrome is associated with an increased risk of early mortality. As you can see, low testosterone is just the tip of the iceberg.

"Just tell me what to do, Doc. Tell me exactly what to do, and I'll do it."

That's what I hear from men every day.

But, what are they really asking for? What they really want to know is:

- Is my testosterone level normal, or not?
- If it is normal, why am I still feeling like a shell of the man I used to be?
- What should I eat? What shouldn't I eat?
- What's the deal with this intermittent fasting thing everyone is talking about these days?
- How do I sleep better?
- How do I manage all the stress in my life?
- What exercises should I be doing? When is the best time to work out? Should I be hitting the gym before I eat or after?
- What supplements should I be taking?

These are all valid questions, and they don't always have a straightforward answer. There's no shortage of information out there, but it can be tough to distinguish the "fake news" from the real deal.

There's even more to it than that. In our society, men are encouraged to work harder and sleep less. They're expected to "hustle." As a result, most run on autopilot. They function every day in survival mode, just trying to stay afloat and get through each day. And when everything inevitably comes crashing down, *that's* when they finally decide to go see a doctor.

This is a big reason why Male 1.0 has failed. And it's time for a replacement that actually works.

As I mentioned earlier, I went through the exact same thing. But my personal interest in finding a solution actually began long before that health crisis in my early forties, and it goes much deeper.

When I was very young, my parents divorced, after which I didn't see much of my father. Through our nearly non-existent relationship, I learned firsthand how important a strong healthy man is to his family and the detrimental effects of his absence.

A few years later, when I was about eight years old, I came to a profound realization: I *knew* that I was born to be a doctor. I became obsessed with learning how the body functions, and I loved the idea of being able to help people get well.

Everything came together years later as I progressed through my medical education. My early childhood experience had taught me the importance of a father to a family. And it motivated me to help men be strong, healthy, and present. I decided the best way for me to do that was to specialize in men's health, which is what ultimately led me to urology.

After years of practice, however, an unfortunate truth became clear to me: men weren't taking care of themselves, and as a result they were failing themselves and their families.

This wasn't their fault, of course; they simply didn't know any other way, as evidenced by the plea – "Just tell me what to do" – that I heard every day in my office. No one talked about resources men could turn to for information or guidance because, until now, there weren't any.

Male 2.0 is more than just another trajectory in my career. It's following through on my commitment to help men optimize their health so they can be powerful and present husbands, fathers and leaders.

You don't have to struggle through each day, just hoping to get by. You don't have to struggle with low energy and feeling like crap. You don't have to live with erectile dysfunction, or low sex drive. No matter your age, you don't have to live like this anymore.

Now, do I have a magic pill like the one Bradley Cooper pops in the movie *Limitless*? Absolutely not, and anyone that promises that is likely being dishonest. I do, however, have real life solutions, and my goal is to share them with as many men as possible.

CHAPTER TWO

LET'S TALK ABOUT SEX, BABY...

Jason couldn't quite look me in the eye. He sat on the exam table, wringing his hands nervously as his gaze darted from the floor to the wall behind me and back again. It was my first time seeing him, so I had no idea what to expect. Finally, and with great hesitation, he began to speak.

"It just keeps happening, Doc. Night after night, I'm letting my wife down."

Jason was in his early forties, but he was already struggling with erectile dysfunction. Erections didn't come easily for him, and his wife saw it as a sign that he was no longer attracted to her. His marriage was unraveling, and Jason saw that appointment with me as a last resort to try to hold things together.

I see young, embarrassed guys like Jason every day. As a urologist who specializes in men's health, I know that men typically come to see me when their favorite organ isn't working properly. It's not the *only* reason of course, but if there's one thing that motivates men most, this is it.

Guys suffer from crappy sleep. They tolerate gaining weight. They even get used to muddling through the day completely exhausted with no energy. But what guys can't live without is sex.

Predictably, Jason asked me for testosterone shots and that "little blue pill." When I told him that neither would solve his problems, he nearly crumbled.

9

"You mean there's no way to fix this?" Jason asked with a good dose of panic in his voice.

This is a good place to hit pause on the story and talk about your body a bit. Think of a fancy sports car, like a Ferrari. If you check out the engine, there are a lot of moving parts. And they all have to be working properly in order for you to take a ride. When one small part stops working, it affects the entire engine, and ultimately, the car's performance.

Jason was obese, with the typical beer belly. When I asked him about his nutrition, he told me that for lunch he usually grabbed fast food or snacks from the vending machine in his office building. For dinner, he and his wife often had frozen prepackaged meals or ordered in pizza. The funny thing was, he actually thought he ate "pretty well"!

He painted an equally unhealthy picture when I asked about his lifestyle. As the head of a division at a huge corporation, his job involved long hours, including weekends. He rarely had time to sit down to a real meal during the day, which explained his poor lunch choices. He had a demanding boss who was never satisfied with anything. It therefore came as no surprise when he revealed that he wasn't sleeping very well and was always stressed. He rarely exercised and had very few leisure activities that he enjoyed.

When I did my usual workup, I found that his testosterone level was low and his blood pressure and cholesterol levels were elevated. His fasting glucose and insulin levels were elevated as well, suggesting insulin resistance — an early indicator of type 2 diabetes. His hsCRP (high-sensitivity C-reactive protein) was elevated, a marker indicative of chronic inflammation, and his cortisol levels — an indicator of chronic stress — were markedly abnormal.

Remember my Ferrari analogy. All of our bodily systems interact together to create a finely tuned machine, so when one system doesn't work there are often several others that don't work either. That means that addressing one system alone will not be helpful; in order to effect real change, we must address *all* of them.

Like so many others, Jason was only focused on a quick fix to his sexual function. But he had much bigger problems. And while it started with low testosterone, that was just the beginning.

He wasn't aware that his sexual issues were closely tied to his blood pressure, high cholesterol, insulin resistance, chronic inflammation, and obesity. All of these factors together provided the underlying basis for his troubles in the bedroom. And it was ALL directly related to his terrible lifestyle — poor nutrition, poor sleep, poor stress management, lack of exercise and social activities.

Erectile dysfunction is a very common motivator for guys to come see me for help. However, it's rarely the *actual* problem, but instead merely a marker of more significant underlying health issues. This is why giving testosterone or the blue pill doesn't help — they simply mask the symptoms.

There are millions of men like Joe, Marty and Jason. They are *real* men who, like you, need *real* solutions.

This is the men's health epidemic, and to overcome it, we need to change the way we live.

We need to upgrade to Male 2.0.

CHAPTER THREE

FIX IT BECAUSE IT IS BROKEN

We need to drastically overhaul our healthcare system. It's reactive medicine, based not on health but on treating disease and managing symptoms. At best, this system aims to keep us in a neutral state — no illness, but no wellness either.

We have been conditioned to buy into this system. We go about our lives with little focus on our health. Then, when we get sick, we go see a doctor, who conducts a handful of tests, diagnoses us with a disease, and sends us on our way with a prescription, or two, or three. We take the medication, feel better, and get back to our lives... and the cycle starts all over again.

The problem is that just because you're not acutely sick does NOT mean that you're healthy. Men go through their lives feeling awful every day thinking it's normal. They don't know any better, and how could they, when the current healthcare model leads us to believe that if you're not "sick" you're perfectly fine?

Why aren't more medical doctors talking about how broken our healthcare system really is? The reason is simple – we've been indoctrinated just like everyone else.

The process of becoming a medical doctor is grueling, rigorous, and brutally exhausting. For as much hell as we put our bodies through during our medical training, it's no wonder we're not being groomed to focus on health!

We are overwhelmed with learning the science as well as the actual clinical practice of treating patients. We often work all day and night, treating sick patients in the hospital, doing everything we can just to keep them alive.

We learn how to treat acute, life-threatening problems and how to manage conditions that often have no cure. We learn the disease model, where we treat symptoms and stamp out disease.

Can you imagine going to see a doctor, not because you're sick but because you want to *optimize your health*? Because you want to be as healthy as humanly possible and feel amazing?

Or how about going to a doctor to learn how to improve the quantity and quality of your sleep? Or what you should eat and when? Or how to mitigate the effects of stress on your life? Or how to incorporate exercise into your busy life, or how to have a healthy mindset? Or how about going to a doctor simply to live longer?

Most doctors wouldn't even know what to do with you if you tried.

The worst part is that we've actually regressed. A lot. Back in ancient times, Hippocrates, who's considered the father of modern medicine, followed a completely different model, one that was centered on the patient rather than disease. In *De Alimento*, he wrote, "In food, excellent medicine can be found; in food, bad medicine can be found…" So you see, the "secret" I'm talking about is nothing new; it's just been forgotten.

According to Hippocrates, health is not merely an absence of disease but a state of dynamic equilibrium between one's internal and external environments. It's a delicate balance, and when it's thrown off, a person becomes ill.

A bit of irony is that all doctors take the Hippocratic Oath prior to starting their careers. Unfortunately, we've become far removed from how Hippocrates envisioned the field of medicine.

So, how do we fix it? We shift the paradigm. We revert back to the way medicine was intended to be practiced. We start by moving towards health and wellness instead of moving away from disease.

We focus on optimized health and peak performance.

We focus on becoming limitless.

This is the Male 2.0 movement.

CHAPTER FOUR

YOUR GENES ARE NOT YOUR DESTINY

For a long time, the prevailing belief was that our fate was tied to our genetics. If your father had a heart attack, it was only a matter of time before you did as well. You could eat well and exercise, but you couldn't outrun your genes.

In recent years we've come to find that this is not the case. The truth is that over 90% of most chronic illnesses are caused, not by genetics, but by environmental factors.

So, what does that actually mean? It means that your health, and risk of illness or disease, is ultimately determined by what you eat, the quality and quantity of your sleep, your fitness, how much stress you experience, environmental exposures, your social connections, and even your mindset.

Do you remember learning about Charles Darwin and natural selection in school? Darwin theorized that organisms change over millions of years due to naturally occurring genetic variations that best allow them to survive and thrive.

For example, it was presumed that the fastest cheetahs were the most adept hunters, so they would be the ones most likely to find food, survive, and reproduce. This explained why cheetahs, as a species, are known for their speed and stealth as predators.

Jean-Baptiste Lamarck, however, had an entirely different theory. He proposed that organisms could change within a generation or two and that, ultimately, animals developed particular traits over the course of their lives based entirely on their interactions with their environment.

The reason you may not have ever heard of Lamarck is that he was considered a quack while Darwin's theory became accepted as scientific gospel. We now know that Lamarck was well ahead of his time because he was absolutely correct. The truth is that your DNA blueprint is significantly affected by external factors that are *absolutely within your control*. This is what we call "epigenetics," which means literally "above the genes."

Simply put, you have more control over your destiny than you realize. Think of it as taking a ride in your Ferrari that I described previously. You were led to believe that you're merely a passenger, and you have to just sit tight, hang on, and try not to get thrown out when the ride gets bumpy. The truth is you can actually take the wheel!

I'll explain, but first it's time for a quiz. These are the leading causes of death in the United States:

- Heart Disease
- Cancer
- Lung Disease
- Accidents
- Stroke

- Alzheimer's Disease
- Diabetes
- Pneumonia / flu
- Kidney Disease
- Suicide

How many of these leading causes of mortality are caused by lifestyle?

If you guessed a few of them, nope! If you guessed most of them, nope again! It may be hard to believe, but ALL of these top ten causes of death in the United States are *directly* related to lifestyle.

This means that YOU directly affect your outcome, not the genes that you're stuck with. You are in the driver's seat of your Ferrari.

With this ability, however, comes responsibility. This means that a lot of your lifestyle habits that you may think are harmless or "not that bad" are negatively affecting your health and longevity.

In the upcoming chapters, you will learn more about how this is entirely within your control. You will learn how you can make changes, starting today, that can expand your human potential beyond what you ever thought possible. You have the power not only to maximize your **LIFESPAN** (how long you live), but your **HEALTHSPAN** (how long you stay healthy).

So, now that I have your attention, let's get down to the details. What exactly is epigenetics, and how can it change your life dramatically from here on out?

Epigenetics is the study of changes in gene expression that do not involve alterations to the actual genetic code. It's the science of how our DNA reacts to its environment.

Now, what does that mean in plain English, Doc?

Every cell in your body has the same genetic code – twenty-three pairs of chromosomes, half of each pair from your mother and the other half from your father .Each chromosome is a long strand of DNA that's arranged as a double helix – like a spiral staircase – and wrapped up and organized around proteins called *histones*. Your DNA is composed of over three billion tiny base pairs that code for your unique genetic blueprint. Functional segments of that strand of DNA are what we call "genes."

Now how does each cell in your body know what to do, or how to function? For example, how does one cell know to become a brain cell while another one becomes a muscle fiber? Remember, each and every cell in your body has the exact same copy of your DNA.

The answer is epigenetics. Complex chemical modifications to your DNA or histones (such as methylation, acetylation, or phosphorrylation, for example) provide signals that tell each gene whether to turn on or turn off. Think of this signaling mechanism as a dimmer switch.

While your genetic code is fixed and never changes (other than rare mutations, which are a whole other topic), the activity of your genes ("genetic expression") varies. This all happens based on epigenetic signals.

So why is any of this important to you? Because gene expression means protein and enzyme production, which is the underlying molecular process for everything that happens in your body.

Your DNA is effectively your hardware, and epigenetics is your software.

Another great analogy is a piano. Every piano has the same keys, and those keys don't ever change. But how those keys are played can make the difference between a bunch of noise and beautiful music.

Epigenetics affects us constantly. It affects our mood and behavior by altering the production of neurotransmitters. Epigenetics affects the way we metabolize food, the way we burn fat, and the way we build muscle. It affects our hormone production and function, as well as DNA repair.

Epigenetics affects cognitive function, memory, and the production of enzymes responsible for metabolism. All of those things together affect our lifespan and healthspan, either by optimizing them or diminishing them, depending entirely on the choices we make.

A study out of Madrid looked at forty sets of identical twins, ranging in age from three to seventy-four. What they found was that the younger twins who shared a similar lifestyle had very similar epigenetic markers on their DNA. But the older twins who had lived apart and had entirely different lifestyles had markedly different epigenetic markers on their DNA. Of course, the twins still shared an identical genome, but their methylation patterns were completely different. What this study demonstrated is that lifestyle and our environment have a critical effect on DNA methylation, and thus gene expression.

It's no longer a question of nature vs. nurture — we know it's a combination of both.

So, what creates these epigenetic signals that affect the function and expression of your genes? The answer: almost everything! This includes what you eat, when you eat, how you sleep, how you move, how you experience stress, how you breathe, and even how you think.

We know that six months of regular exercise increases the positive expression of nearly seven thousand genes. That's nearly 30% of our entire genome! And just one night of poor sleep negatively affects the function of our "clock" genes, which produce enzymes critical for numerous bodily functions regulated by our circadian rhythms (our internal sleep and awake cycle). Makes you think twice about one night of less-than-stellar sleep, doesn't it? These are just two examples and I could go on, but you get the idea.

It's critical to understand that each of us responds very differently to our environment based on our unique genetics.

This explains why the fad diet that made one guy lose fifty pounds did nothing for another guy, other than raise his cholesterol. And it explains why you may be a natural night owl who does better by staying up late and sleeping late, while someone else may need to be in bed by nine p.m. in order to function well the next day.

Simply stated, your genotype (genes), together with epigenetics (your environment and lifestyle) equals your phenotype (you!). More about this later...

CHAPTER FIVE

WHAT IS MALE 2.0?

et's return now to Joe, Marty and Jason. They each came to me for different reasons, but they were all looking for a boost in testosterone. They were convinced that a virile man-potion would solve all their problems. And why wouldn't they think that? Testosterone has been touted as the magical solution to all men's health issues, especially as they age. The problem with this approach is that restoring and optimizing men's health is so much more complex than just increasing one hormone.

You may think it's all about testosterone, but it's not. While it starts with T, it never ends there.

What do I mean by that? Well, there's no question that testosterone is the juice that keeps a man running at an optimal level. It's the power source that keeps the human male version of the Energizer Bunny going and going and going. That said, focusing solely on testosterone as a cure-all is missing the bigger picture.

Remember the Ferrari analogy. Testosterone may be the gas that fuels it. But to get your finely-tuned machine operating at its peak – so you can lose weight, build muscle, have better sex, think better, live longer, and feel amazing – you have to consider every moving part in the system.

In my early days as a doctor, when guys like Joe came to me for treatment, I dutifully gave them a shot of testosterone and sent them on their way. What I started to notice was that some guys improved on this treatment while others didn't, regardless of how their testosterone levels responded.

The ones that got better on testosterone shots showed up for their regular doses, happy as can be. But I didn't know how to help the ones who weren't happy, the ones who were still suffering, the ones who didn't get anywhere on this treatment. I didn't know how to make them better because despite years of intense, hands-on education, I hadn't learned any other options myself.

I had not yet developed Male 2.0 ...

In order to explain what Male 2.0 is, I must first tell you what it's NOT.

Male 2.0 is NOT a gimmick or some kind of new drug or fad diet. It doesn't include the "limitless" pill or a miracle solution that's going to magically make all your problems go away.

Male 2.0 is NOT something you can buy and have it do all the work for you.

Male 2.0 is NOT reactive; nor is it a band-aid for your symptoms or treatment of a disease.

Male 2.0 is also NOT about simply eating more vegetables and exercising. You already know that and you certainly don't need this book to tell you.

Most importantly, Male 2.0 is NOT a one-size-fits-all, "perfect" diet or exercise program (because there isn't one). It's not cookie-cutter because YOU aren't.

So, what is Male 2.0?

Male 2.0 is taking full ownership of your life and your health.

Male 2.0 is a transformation. It's living with intention. It's upgrading to the most amazing, optimized version of yourself. It's about unleashing your full inner potential.

Male 2.0 is about becoming more than just a man ... it empowers you to be THE MAN.

Male 2.0 is no longer waiting until you're sick to seek out medical guidance. It's proactive and preventative. It's about getting behind the wheel of your Ferrari and taking control.

Male 2.0 is changing your entire approach to your health and your life. It's about being laser-focused on your "Big Why" so that everything you do is in alignment.

Male 2.0 is data-driven. Every decision you make about your health is based on real-life data. No more guessing. If you can track it, you can manage it.

Male 2.0 is based on precision medicine. Instead of a one-size-fits-all approach to health, it's personalized, based on your unique genetic blueprint.

Male 2.0 is not merely an adjustment to your lifestyle, but a sustainable change in how you live and how you think.

Male 2.0 is ultimately a movement, focused on overcoming the men's health epidemic and shifting the paradigm of men's health.

When you upgrade to Male 2.0, you'll feel like a man again. You'll feel like you're back in your prime — with high energy, a great sex drive, and confidence in your appearance. And you'll perform in the bedroom like you did in your twenties. You'll feel alive again.

And once you live the Male 2.0 lifestyle, you'll realize that it's not so complicated at all. The only regret you may have is that you didn't know about it sooner.

Here's the thing — when they told you that it's all just a normal part of aging, they LIED. And when they told you it can all be fixed with a testosterone shot, they lied again.

I want to reiterate that, yes, testosterone absolutely is crucial for maintaining men's health. That said, testosterone therapy on its own is not going to fix your underlying problems because it doesn't get to the root of the problem. It's one hormone, albeit a critical one, that interacts closely with others such as cortisol, thyroid hormone, estrogen, growth hormone, and insulin (yes, insulin is a hormone).

All of these hormones need to work together in a perfect balance to create optimal health. And this can all be drastically affected by your nutrition, your sleep, your micronutrient levels, your stress levels, your breathing, and so much more, including how you think.

So you can see how your "Ferrari" needs a lot more than just gas. It can't operate at its peak if every single part of the system is not working perfectly. This is why we take what's called a *systems-based approach*, and we do so through the lens of your unique genetic blueprint.

Before I dig too deeply into the details of Male 2.0, I want you to ask yourself these questions:

- How much do you want your life to change?
- How badly do you want to feel like a man again?
- How badly do you want to feel amazing?
- What are you willing to do to make that happen?

Are you willing to become intentional with everything you do and take responsibility for your health?

Are you willing to put down the junk food and start eating better?

Are you willing to get up off the couch and exercise?

Are you willing to give up late nights so you can get a good night's sleep every night?

Are you ready to improve your performance at work, at play, and in the bedroom?

Are you ready to start operating at your peak, like you did years or even decades ago?

If so, keep reading because I have lots to tell you.

When you upgrade to Male 2.0, you will be the best version of yourself. As strong as you can be. As well-rested as you can be. At the healthiest weight you can be, and with low risk for chronic disease. And, ultimately, as confident and empowered as you can be.

What that means is that you're not merely going through the motions of life in a reactive state. You're not just waiting for the next disaster or health issue to arise.

It's about precision.

It's about making a decision.

It's about living with intention to reach a state of peak performance.

It's about becoming limitless.

So, how do you upgrade to Male 2.0? Let's dive in.

CHAPTER SIX

THE MALE 2.0 METHOD

By this point you're probably thinking, *Sounds great, Doc, but what exactly do I do?*

Okay, here goes...

Male 2.0 has four main components:

M = Mindset

A = Aging

L = Lifestyle

E = Environment

We're going to dive deep into each of these components of the Male 2.0 Method, but first here's a brief overview...

To upgrade to Male 2.0, we attack **Mindset** as the first order of business. This is not merely because it's the first letter in the acronym, but because if your mind isn't in the right place, you're not going to be focused and you're not going to invest the energy and grit needed to do everything else.

I'll go into more detail about mindset and overcoming limiting beliefs soon. Just know that this is something I've found to be critical for guys like you who wanted to feel like a man again, feel like themselves again, and live life to its fullest. You can't do any of that if you don't completely believe it's possible, so getting your head on straight is job one.

Next, we look at reversing the processes of **Aging**. It's been assumed that aging is inevitable. Yes, we do get older, there's no way around that. That said, we don't have to get *old*. Research suggests that aging is a "dis-ease" that can be treated. There are cutting-edge approaches that have actually been shown to not only slow aging but actually *reverse* the aging process.

Then we'll spend time focused on **Lifestyle** choices. How is the way you're going about life taking away from your lifespan and healthspan? A huge part of it is nutrition, and not just *what* you're eating, but *when*. We'll dig deep into the mistakes guys make by taking on the latest fad diet, and why it works for some while ruining the health of others.

We'll also get into exercise — which forms are best for you, how exercise affects the other systems in your body, and the best way to incorporate exercise into your life. This lifestyle component also includes stress management and improving both the quantity and quality of your sleep, because both of those are absolutely crucial for your health.

And lastly, we will address **Environmental exposures**. You have no idea how toxicants (called endocrine disruptors) in the products you use every single day are crushing you — including your testosterone levels, fertility, metabolism, and more. We'll focus on how to eliminate exposure to these toxicants and improve your body's ability to overcome their effects.

Now I want to emphasize a critical aspect of applying each of the steps of the Male 2.0 Method: epigenetics and precision medicine. What that means is that optimizing your health and performance is largely done by customization.

Remember our earlier discussion about epigenetics, or gene expression. Epigenetic signals, such as your nutrition, your sleep, or toxicants in your personal care products have the power to turn genes in every cell of your body on and off, like a dimmer switch.

To be more specific, your genetics play a huge role in this process. What I mean is that each of you respond to these epigenetic signals differently based on your genetics.

For example, some people may lose weight with a diet high in complex carbs, whereas others need to eat a low-carb diet to lose weight. Or, if your genetics suggest that you're at high risk for Alzheimer's Disease, we can make precise changes in your diet and lifestyle to specifically lower that risk.

This personalization is a critical aspect of the Male 2.0 Method. We're not just focused on simply eating more veggies and exercising more. That's old school.

Male 2.0 is centered around individualization of your health. It's about precision. And we're going to take a very different approach from the disease-oriented model that currently dominates health-care.

It's not just about treating symptoms or stamping out disease. The goal is total optimization, so you're thriving, not merely surviving.

With each of my concierge clients, I develop a comprehensive, customized precision performance plan based on their unique genetic blueprint. In this book, however, I'm going to arm you with enough information to start implementing the Male 2.0 Method on your own — *today*.

Be sure to check out drtracygapin.com/book for the FREE Male 2.0 Guide that includes specific tips, tools and cheat sheets mentioned in the coming chapters. You'll also learn how you can leverage your genetic blueprint to optimize your health and reverse aging. I promise that your vitality will improve just from making small incremental changes to your daily routine.

Now get ready, because we're going to dive deep into each of the components of the Male 2.0 Method.

CHAPTER SEVEN

IT'S ALL IN YOUR HEAD (MINDSET)

Let's get real for a moment — no one likes to hear that something is "all in your head;" however, like most clichés, this one holds quite a bit of truth. If your thoughts, beliefs and focus are not in the right place, you're never going to succeed. Not at work, not in your personal life, and most certainly not on your health journey.

You know how some people are always trying to lose weight, while for others the pounds seem to come right off? That's not because of a fancy diet plan, or because they managed to magically fire up their metabolism all of a sudden.

It's because a decision was made. That's how every victory begins — with an empowering decision that led to a commitment, that ultimately led to success.

The first step in the Male 2.0 Method is MINDSET because it's where everything starts. No man can transform his life and his health without getting into the right frame of mind.

Now, take this moment to ask yourself:

Are you truly committed to doing everything you need to do to transform your health and your life?

Are you ready to take your health seriously and make it a priority?

Are you ready to change the way you're doing life?

Are you ready to change your daily habits?

I get it — change can be difficult. The status quo – as undesirable as it may be — is familiar and comfortable. But if you want to upgrade to Male 2.0, you must make the decision to leave comfort behind and step onto a new path.

Why must this be a conscious decision? Because one of the most powerful aspects of this transformation is *living with intention.* This means that everything you do, every choice you make, is purposeful, precise, and in alignment with your goals.

It All Starts with Your "*WHY*"

Take a moment to consider your reasons for undertaking this transformation.

Is it for your kids, so that you can have more energy and stamina to play with them?

Is it for your wife, so that you can reliably satisfy her?

Is it for yourself, so that you can get more out of life? Or feel confident about how you look and feel?

You don't have to limit it to one reason, but you do have to be very clear on exactly *why* you're doing this.

Why is your WHY so important? Because changing your eating habits, developing a consistent exercise program, altering your sleep schedule, and confronting the stress in your life isn't going to be easy.

There will be times when you're tempted to give up – times when you just want to grab a donut, skip the gym and stay up all night binge-watching your favorite Netflix shows. At these times, your WHY will be the motivator that keeps you on track.

So take some time right now to nail down your *WHY.* Write it down and put it on your nightstand. Then take out your phone and take a picture of it.

Every morning when you wake up, the very first thing you need to do is read your *WHY* out loud.

Every night when you go to bed, the very last thing you need to do is read your *WHY* out loud.

Several times a day, look at that picture on your phone and read your *WHY* out loud.

This reminder will not only keep you on track so you make better choices in the moment; it will also retrain your brain, become a part of your new, heathier mindset, and help you live with intention.

Finally, your WHY will be a driving factor for two components that are critical for success as you embark on your new health journey — accountability and motivation.

Limiting Beliefs

The next aspect of mindset we need to address is limiting beliefs. As the name suggests, these are beliefs that place a cap on what you can achieve.

You will never achieve what you don't believe is possible for you. Therefore, in order to transform your health, you have to change your beliefs around health.

We have already discussed epigenetics, whereby your genes are constantly switched on or off depending on your thoughts, feelings, and emotions. In addition, studies show that your thoughts alone are capable of expanding your cognitive and physical performance. As award-winning journalist and author Lynne McTaggart wrote in her book, *The Intention Experiment*, "Every thought we have is tangible energy with the power to transform."

Limiting beliefs are a common obstacle on our path to success, not only with regard to health but in all areas of life. How many limiting beliefs have you felt at some point?

Some examples:

"I'm not [good, smart, strong, talented] enough."

"I could never do that."

"I'm too old."

"There's nothing I can do about my [health, diet, fitness]."

"I might do it wrong."

"There's not enough time."

"I don't know where to start."

"I don't have the skillset."

"I don't have the money."

"I can't change."

I'm sure you can think of many more. These limiting beliefs are ingrained, unconscious patterns in your mind that are holding you back from reaching your full human potential.

Limiting beliefs are not real, but myths, usually based on false perceptions stemming from a prior bad experience. When we accept these myths as fact, we experience life through their faulty lens and our brain consistently finds evidence in our everyday reality to support them. We give them the power to destroy our joy and keep us from having what we want.

To overcome this, you first need to notice your limiting beliefs, then create new empowering beliefs to replace them. This is the power of the mind. The power of decision.

Take a moment to list all of your limiting beliefs. Why are you not where you want to be? What's holding you back from reaching your goals?

Once you've created an exhaustive list, read through each reason, and then ask yourself why you believe that to be true. Did it originate with you, or is it something someone else told you? You may be surprised to find that most of your limiting beliefs have been imposed upon you, and you subconsciously accepted them as truth.

Now cross out each of those limiting beliefs and write down the empowering beliefs that replace them and support your upgrade to Male 2.0.

Some examples:

"I am [good, smart, strong, talented] enough."

"I could absolutely do that."

"I'm never too old."

"There's so much I can do to improve and optimize my [health, diet, fitness]."

"I will learn how to do it right!"

"There's always enough time."

"I can figure out where to start."

"I have the skills, or else I can learn them."

"I have enough money."

"I am flexible enough to change."

Now I want you to write these down and read them aloud every single morning when you wake up and every night before you go to bed.

You have to change the way you see yourself, your worth, your value, and your truly limitless potential.

Gratitude

One last key piece of the mindset component of Male 2.0 is gratitude. When you cultivate an attitude of gratitude, you are choosing to feel thankful for what you have, are, and experience. Over time, this attitude can become your default state of mind and a powerful magnet, attracting more of what you want into your life.

Research has shown that gratitude has a significant impact on both your physical and mental health. It causes a surge in rewarding neurotransmitters such as dopamine and reduces depression and fatigue.

It's also associated with reduced biomarkers of inflammation, improved heart rate variability (a precise physiologic indicator of your health — more on this later!), and better quality and quantity of sleep. Gratitude also keeps you grounded with a constant reminder of what's important and what isn't.

For example, when things go wrong at work, instead of getting upset, stop and take a moment to be grateful. Be grateful that you have a job! And be grateful for your healthy children, loving wife, and everything else that's precious to you.

By focusing on what you're grateful for, you put things into proper perspective. You can then ask yourself if whatever made you mad truly matters, and if it's worth a shred of your energy. At that point, the trivial stuff just fades away.

I want you to try a *thirty-day gratitude challenge*. Every night before you go to bed, write down five things you're thankful for. When you wake up in the morning, I want you to read your list from the night before.

Refocusing on the positives will retrain your mind to not to get upset when it's not worth it, and instead focus on what really matters — your *WHY*.

We can't control a lot of what happens in our lives, but we absolutely can control our thoughts. Once you master that, you become unstoppable. Limitless. And where your mind goes, your body ultimately follows...

Remember to check out the FREE Male 2.0 Guide at drtracygapin.com/book for specific tools related to optimizing mindset!

Let's look at the next part of the Male 2.0 Method — reversing the aging process.

CHAPTER EIGHT

TICK TOCK (AGING)

C onventional wisdom tells us that aging is inevitable; it's just something that happens outside of our control. But what if everything we were led to believe was wrong? What if aging is a disease that could be treated? What if we could not only slow aging, but actually reverse it? The good news is we can, and that's why AGING is the second component of the Male 2.0 Method.

In order to fight aging, we need to first understand how it happens. We need to identify which systems are involved, and how we can optimize them to work in our favor.

People may tell you aging is all about testosterone. Remember that it may start there, but certainly doesn't end there!

As you probably already know, we're made up of cells — around thirty trillion or so to be precise. Over time, our cells stop working as efficiently as they did when we were younger.

Most people think of aging as what you can see — grey hair, wrinkles, a beer gut, et cetera. But the truth is that the gradual decline in function we're concerned with is happening on a cellular level, hence the term "cellular aging." It's this underlying process that we must address in order to not just slow down aging, but actually reverse it.

Hallmarks of Cellular Aging

There are several known hallmarks of cellular aging. It's beyond the scope of this book to dive deep into the science of each of them — I'll save that for the next one! But it's important for the sake of this discussion to understand some of the key underlying aging processes that we want to impact.

These theories about the underlying causes of cellular aging are all supported by extensive research and science. Don't be discouraged as we go through them, because later we're going to talk about exactly how to address and reverse each one.

Let's start with garbage...

Autophagy

One of the most amazing things about our cells is that when we're young, they're basically "self-cleaning." What do I mean by that? They actually have a system for getting rid of waste, kind of like a garbage disposal.

Cells contain structures called lysosomes which act as the cell's digestive system. The lysosomes in your cells spend their time breaking down cellular material, recycling what your body can use and degrading the junk. This process is called *autophagy*, and when we're young our cells are experts at it. Our lysosomes work like tireless conveyor belts, clearing out waste and keeping our cells operating at their fullest potential.

As we age, the process of autophagy slows down, or sometimes fails altogether, effectively turning our cells into hoarders. Just like you can't function well when you're surrounded by garbage, neither can your cells.

One of the ways we can fight aging is to jumpstart, or at least encourage, autophagy in our cells.

Telomeres

Next is telomere shortening. Remember your chromosomes and the DNA double helix I spoke about earlier in this book? Well, your DNA has end caps called telomeres. Think of them as the plastic tips on shoelaces. What would happen if your shoelaces didn't have those? They'd fray and unravel, and your shoelace would quickly cease to be functional.

Similarly, as your cells replicate and age over time, your telomeres get worn out and shorten. As they shorten, they lose their ability to adequately protect your DNA, which can lead to DNA damage and instability and ultimately faulty cellular function. Your cells get damaged and lose their ability to divide and replicate and your body can no longer regenerate any new healthy cells. Hello, aging.

Senescence

Over time, cellular damage can lead to the accumulation of toxic *"senescent"* cells. Senescent cells are old, worthless and functionally inactive, which is why they are often referred to as "zombie cells." They also secrete toxins that actually damage nearby normal healthy cells, so protecting your telomeres and clearing senescent cells is a huge priority.

Mitochondria

Now let's look at the *mitochondria*, the powerhouse of every cell. Think of the mitochondria like the cell's engines, utilizing micro-nutrients and a magic molecule called NAD^+ to create an essential form of energy called adenosine triphosphate (ATP). ATP is the powerful energy supply that drives every single function in your body.

As we age, our NAD+ levels diminish and our mitochondria become dysfunctional. They lose the ability to efficiently provide the critical ATP that we need to thrive. When this happens, we start showing signs of aging with declining energy, muscle tone, and exercise capacity. Therefore, one key approach to reversing aging is to optimize mitochondrial function.

This starts with maintaining healthy levels of NAD+, although there has been some debate about the best way to do this. Intermittent fasting and exercise have been shown to increase NAD+ levels. There are also several supplements that include pre-cursors of NAD+, including nicotinamide riboside (NR) and nicotinamide mononucleotide (NMN). Studies are ongoing to determine the most effective approach.

Protein Cross-linking

A key process of aging is *protein cross-linking*. This means that proteins get bound by other molecules, causing them to not function properly. The most common culprit for this is sugar.

In a process called glycation, excess sugar in your bloodstream and tissues binds to critical proteins and enzymes to create what are called advanced glycation end-products (AGEs). These AGEs plug up the normal machinery of your cells, wreak havoc on your system, and ultimately promote aging.

Therefore, one of the key approaches to reversing aging is to prevent cross-linking through tight glucose regulation. This means consistently maintaining optimal blood sugar levels.

Programmed Aging

Another important theory of aging is *"programmed aging"* – in other words, that the human body is simply designed to age. This suggests that certain genes are intentionally switched on or off as we age.

A critical gene called AMPK (AMP-activated protein kinase) and a family of genes called the sirtuins are genes that "turn off" as you age. Another gene called mTOR (mammalian target of rapamycin) promotes aging by turning "on." Addressing the expression of these genes is a key focus in age management.

All of these are aspects of aging that we can not only slow down, but actually reverse. As we go through the rest of this book, we're going to talk about exactly how you can do that.

Endocrine Theory

Finally, there is the endocrine theory of aging — the concept that changes in hormone production and function is what ultimately controls the aging process. Let's spend a moment and examine how your hormones, especially testosterone, fit into the big picture of optimizing health and reversing the aging process.

CHAPTER NINE

RAGING HORMONES (AGING)

J ake sat on the exam table, staring at me hopefully. He didn't beat around the bush.

"I need a testosterone shot, Doc."

Here we go again... but wait. I suspected that there was something more here than the typical low testosterone story.

Jake was a sluggish five-foot-nine and two hundred twenty-five pounds. He told me he was always cold, and in fact, he was wearing a sweater and pants in the middle of July. If you've ever been to Sarasota, Florida in the middle of summer you would think twice about that outfit.

Jake described how he had constant brain fog and difficulty focusing at work. He was always tired and ran out of energy halfway through the day. He was also depressed and unmotivated to get back in the gym.

When I looked at Jake's lab results, I could see that his testosterone levels were indeed quite low. But that wasn't his only problem.

His thyroid levels were really low, too. And his afternoon cortisol (stress hormone) levels were super low, suggesting chronic physiologic stress and/or inflammation. His insulin and hemoglobin A1c levels were high, indicating insulin resistance, which is an early sign of diabetes.

Jake didn't just need his testosterone fixed. He needed to get his thyroid function back to normal. He needed to deal with chronic inflammation. He needed to get his serum glucose levels under better control. He basically needed a full body overhaul.

He needed what we call a systems-based approach, focusing on every aspect of his health. His issues went far beyond testosterone. As mentioned earlier, testosterone is only one hormone men have to worry about.

Remember how I said that it starts with T, but it never ends there? Simply put, you may think that since you're a man, fixing your testosterone is all you need to do. But that simply isn't true.

Our hormones are like instruments in a symphony, working closely in concert with each other. If any instrument is out of tune, think of how bad the music will sound. To reach and maintain peak performance, we must focus on optimizing all of your hormones.

For example, think of thyroid and testosterone as a couple of buddies holding hands. When one drops, the other drops with it, and they can both hit rock bottom at the same time. I see guys all the time who are suffering with what seems to be low testosterone but are in fact dealing with symptoms related to hypothyroidism (low thyroid function).

Another crucial hormone is cortisol. If you've developed that fatty tire around your waist, chances are good that cortisol is the culprit. What's cortisol, you ask? Well, you may have heard of it referred to as the "stress hormone."

Cortisol is a hormone made by your adrenal gland that, along with adrenaline, helps you rise to the occasion in times of stress. This is known as the "fight or flight" response, which occurs when we perceive ourselves to be in imminent danger. You may know the feeling — your heart races, you start breathing fast, and your throat closes up. Here's the problem — this reaction was very valuable to our Neanderthal ancestors when they were being chased by tigers. They literally needed this to survive.

In this day and age, men no longer have to run from wild animals to stay alive, yet they are accustomed to feeling under attack all the time. We're trying to meet a deadline. We're trying to please a customer or a client. We're expected to work long hours at work, be reliable providers, and care for and protect our family.

Herein lies the problem. Our body doesn't distinguish between the hungry tiger and the demands of modern life, which means when we're continually stressed. And what do we get for it? Chronically altered cortisol levels which leads to elevated blood glucose levels, fat storage, slowed metabolism, and depressed testosterone levels. They are all intimately tied together.

Cortisol is also the currency of chronic inflammation, which has been considered a key underlying root cause of most chronic illness, cancer, as well as the aging processes discussed in Chapter 8.

There are two types of inflammation — acute and chronic. Acute inflammation is your body's natural mounted response to something that has gone wrong, such as an injury or an infection. White blood cells secrete cytokines (pro-inflammatory enzymes) to get rid of toxins and help your body repair damaged tissue, then the inflammatory response fades. This is a good thing.

With chronic inflammation, however, the cytokines don't go away when the acute insult has cleared. The inflammatory response persists, ultimately affecting healthy tissue and organs as well. Think of it as getting hit by friendly fire in the battle of your body.

A key part of the hormone symphony, therefore, is managing cortisol levels and eliminating chronic inflammation.

Another critical hormone to focus on is insulin. You may know about insulin as it relates to diabetes, but it's not black or white. People aren't just healthy or diabetic.

Insulin is created in response to elevated glucose in your blood. It's insulin's job to get your blood sugar level back down to a normal level.

With excess blood sugar, chronic inflammation, stress, or obesity, your insulin levels rise. Over time, however, your cells eventually stop responding to insulin and they can't take in any more sugar. Think of it as needing a place to stay on vacation, but there are no more hotel rooms.

This is called insulin resistance, which leads to overproduction of insulin, more obesity, and the beginning of a very vicious cycle.

The key takeaway here is that each of these hormones interact together in a finely-tuned manner. As an example, let's look at the effects of stress.

Chronic physiologic stress leads to elevated cortisol levels and chronic inflammation. This causes increased serum glucose levels, which leads to increased insulin levels, slowed metabolism and fat storage. This results in lowered testosterone and thyroid hormone levels, which furthers the cycle.

As you can see, you have to approach it all as a complex system. And to optimize your system — achieve peak health, look great, and feel amazing — you can't just look at just testosterone levels. Remember the symphony — every instrument counts!

Let's go back to Jake for a moment. We discovered he had low testosterone, but he also had depressed thyroid function. His cortisol function was abnormal, and he showed signs of chronic inflammation and insulin resistance. I was able to help him by approaching every aspect of his health with a systems-based approach.

When we got his hormones in balance, his brain fog and depression lifted. His energy level improved and he got back in the gym. His sexual vitality returned. He felt like himself again. Once we got to that point, Jake told me that he couldn't remember the last time he felt so good. Isn't that what all men (and women) strive for? To feel good?

The point here is that your body is an intricate web of systems, and your hormone levels all have to be in the zone for you to feel optimized. If you're going to focus solely on your testosterone levels while ignoring all your other hormonal functions, you'll be like that proverbial dog chasing its tail.

But let's get back to testosterone for a moment...

Let me tell you one of the most important things you NEED to know about testosterone but have probably never heard before. It's about how testosterone is measured, and it makes ALL the difference!

There are two levels of testosterone that can be measured when doing diagnostics — *total testosterone* and *free testosterone*. Free testosterone is the bioavailable form, meaning that it's the kind that your body can actually use.

Your free testosterone is unbound to any serum proteins, so it's available to enter the cell, specifically the nucleus, where it works its magic to provide the fuel to power you up as a man. Any testosterone that *is* bound to proteins in the blood — especially SHBG (serum hormone binding globulin) — cannot enter the cell and is thus unable to have any major effect.

Here's where the problem comes in. It's totally possible, and quite common, for your total testosterone to be in the normal range while your free testosterone is low. The big problem is that most doctors don't know about this and *don't even measure free testosterone*. Your doctor will get the results of your total testosterone level and tell you it looks fine and you've got nothing to worry about.

This would be great news, except you still feel like crap, with low energy and mental fog. You're still gaining weight and can't build any muscle. You still have poor libido and issues performing in the bedroom. And you still have issues with cortisol, thyroid hormone, insulin levels, glucose levels, and chronic inflammation.

Again, the *free testosterone* is what matters — not the total testosterone. The free testosterone is the level you need to improve in order to get on the right track toward optimizing your health. Remember, though, that *it starts with T but it doesn't end there.*

Running out to your local testosterone clinic for a T shot is NOT the answer!

Free testosterone is just one part of the systems-based approach to men's health. We have to optimize all of your hormones. And your mindset. And your nutrition, sleep, fitness, and detox systems. But I'm getting ahead of myself...

Now that you have an idea of what happens as you age, let's turn our focus to the good news. All of these issues can be addressed and counteracted at the cellular level using the Male 2.0 Method. Specifically, we are able to:

- Improve autophagy
- Protect your DNA
- Clear senescent cells
- Maximize mitochondrial function
- Eliminate chronic inflammation
- Reduce protein cross-linking

In case you're wondering, yes, this book will walk you through what you can do on a daily basis to reverse these underlying causes of aging. That said...

I must remind you here about epigenetics and the personalized strategies, based on your unique genetics, that can help fine-tune your approach to the Male 2.0 Method. Simply put, once we have a working knowledge of your hardware (your DNA), we can leverage the right software (lifestyle, environment, etc.) to have the desired outcome.

For example, your genetics may point to a predisposition for poor mitochondrial function. This would suggest that we need to place a priority on specific approaches to optimizing mitochondrial health.

Or your genetics may suggest that your thyroid hormone functions normally throughout your body but not so well in your brain. This would potentially cause symptoms of hypothyroidism (low thyroid), even though your serum thyroid hormone levels may be normal. In this case we would focus on specifically increasing thyroid hormone levels in your brain and assessing your response. For others, autophagy or chronic inflammation may be the chief issue to address. This is how we use epigenetics and precision medicine to take a personalized approach to reversing the aging process.

Remember to check out drtracygapin.com/book for the FREE Male 2.0 Guide that has specific tools related to age reversal. You'll also learn how you can work with me and my team to leverage your genetic blueprint to optimize your hormones and reverse aging.

CHAPTER TEN

YOU ARE WHAT YOU EAT (LIFESTYLE)

f I asked you to guess what the leading risk factor for death is in nearly every country on earth, what would your first guess be? (Hint: the title of this chapter gives it away). According to an April 2019 article in *The Lancet* medical journal[1], nothing is more threatening to good health – indeed, to life itself – than poor nutrition.

The bad news is that we're literally eating ourselves to death as a species and show no signs of slowing down. But the good news is that your diet is 100 percent within your control, so this is a risk you can mitigate with some guidance I'll be laying out in this chapter.

First, let me tell you about Eric, a forty-six-year old concierge client of mine from Houston. Eric travelled to his appointment with me the same way he did everything else – in great style, from the private jet he flew to Florida right down to the chauffeured car he took to my office. He was insanely successful as a wealth advisor, but in every other way, Eric was failing.

He wasn't obese but he certainly wasn't in good shape either, as evidenced by the "beer belly" typical of so many men struggling with their health.

Eric was dealing with a lot of cognitive issues, especially mind fog and difficulty concentrating, that were affecting his work with his clients. He told me he wasn't exercising very much because of his busy schedule. And he was depressed and not sleeping well.

Indeed, he looked so tired that he eerily reminded me of my sleepless nights as a surgical intern.

I asked Eric to share details about what he ate, and suddenly everything became clear. Like many busy professionals, Eric didn't make time for meals, let alone to plan healthy ones. Instead, he ate while he worked, around the time and location of meetings, and often settling for fast food or whatever takeout food his staff was ordering that day. His approach to food was not proactive, it was reactive.

He admitted he didn't give much thought to what he ate. He knew he was supposed to eat "healthy," whatever *that* meant. There's so much conflicting information out there, he didn't know what to believe.

I knew that if Eric was going to optimize his health and have any sort of quality of life, he'd need a major overhaul of his eating habits.

Now, let me make one thing clear before we dig too deeply into this topic: *There is no perfect diet.*

The keto diet works well for some people, while it does nothing for others. The same goes for every other diet out there. You know why? If you've been paying attention, your mind should automatically go to that word I keep repeating — epigenetics.

Why is epigenetics a factor here? Because we are all genetically wired to respond differently to various foods; therefore, different diets will affect us in very different ways.

Better stated, there are genes that dictate how we respond to food intake. Let me explain what I mean by that.

We have genes related to our sense of hunger and lack of satiety. Satiety is the sense of feeling full so you can stop eating. You know what I mean – when you're hungry you feel like you can eat everything in sight. But as you eat you start feeling full until you reach the point where you cannot take another bite.

This is the internal thermostat that tells us when we are hungry and when we are full. That figurative threshold for when we are full is different for everyone and, believe it or not, there's a science behind why that happens.

We also have hormones that are directly related to hunger and our sense of satiety. Specifically, the hormones ghrelin and growth hormone tend to promote hunger, whereas the hormones leptin and adiponectin tend to promote the sense of satiety.

We all have an FTO gene, often referred to as the "fat gene" because it's a fat mass and obesity-associated protein. Specifically, it regulates the production of ghrelin.

Some people have a variant of the FTO gene, which can cause them to overeat because their body does not sense that they're full. They're ghrelin levels don't come down like they should when they eat. These people are at an increased risk for obesity, diabetes, chronic inflammation, and other chronic disease that are connected to overeating.

That morbidly obese guy you see stuffing his face at the buffet may in fact have a variant of the FTO gene, making him predisposed to overeating. And if you happen to *be* that guy without a master switch telling you to stop eating, this is all very valuable information indeed.

Why? Because we can make specific changes that address our unique, individual issues, such as taking supplements, focusing on certain foods that are best for our body, or other behavioral modifications.

There are even genes related to snacking and sugar addiction. You know how some people can open a bag of chocolates, eat one or two, and then put the bag away while others eat the whole bag? Well, you can stop blaming it (completely) on a lack of willpower, because there is a genetic factor driving that behavior.

At the end of the book, I'll share with you how you can get your genetic profile done so you'll know if you're a one-or-two-chocolate person or one who shouldn't even reach for the bag.

Learning about your genetics will also explain things like why your neighbor lost weight like crazy on the keto diet and you gained five pounds. Again, this goes back to epigenetics. Specifically, there are genes related to your body's response to carbohydrate intake.

Keep in mind that when I say carbohydrates, I'm talking about complex carbs like leafy greens and sweet potatoes, not simple carbs like donuts and pasta, which most of us know to stay away from.

There's one gene called PLIN-1 (perilipin-1) that's specifically related to the effect of carbohydrate intake on weight loss. Some people's PLIN-1 gene makes them best-suited to lose weight on a high-carb diet, while others will do better with a low-carb diet. Therefore, the PLIN-1 gene can serve as a general guide for how much carbs should be in your diet in order for you to lose weight and build muscle.

There are also genes related to the effect of fat intake on your health. One gene, APOE (Apolipoprotein E), is specifically associated with your body's metabolism of saturated fat, which is found in red meat and dairy products.

Some people do fine with saturated fats, as long as it's in fairly low to moderate amounts. But others who have a variant of the APOE gene have greatly increased risk of developing Alzheimer's disease and cardiovascular disease with saturated fat intake.

As you can see, it's pretty important to know your "APOE status" when deciding whether or not to try a Paleo or keto diet that may be high in saturated fat! This is the power of epigenetics.

There are people with a variant of the APOA (ApolipoproteinA) gene who don't metabolize the polyunsaturated fats in nuts very well and gain weight with them. Others do fine with nuts.

You didn't think protein would be left out of this, did you? Yep, there are genes that regulate how well you metabolize protein.

Some people do great on a high protein diet, while others do very poorly. We've all heard about foods (i.e. turkey) that make us sleepy, but did you know that some people find it hard to fall asleep after eating certain foods?

There's a family of genes called the GAD-1 (Glutamate Decarb-oxylase 1) genes that can have such an effect. The GAD-1 genes are responsible for breaking down the amino acid glutamate that's found in grains and proteins in your diet. This is important because glutamate is a very excitatory neurotransmitter — it stimulates your brain.

The GAD-1 genes help convert glutamate into GABA, which is a very *inhibitory* neurotransmitter. It shuts off your brain's mental spin cycle so you can sleep.

When you eat foods that are high in glutamate, such as grains, eggs, chicken, and MSG, you depend on your GAD-1 genes to do their job so those foods don't turn you into an insomniac. Some people, however, have variants of the GAD-1 genes, and they don't break down glutamate into GABA like they should.

So what should those people do? They should avoid foods that contain glutamate late in the day and at dinnertime so it doesn't affect their sleep. This is epigenetics.

By now I hope you can understand why there's no perfect diet! And you can surely see the value of getting your genetic profile done to learn what foods you should eat, which foods you should avoid, and important risk factors when it comes to your nutrition.

As I mentioned back in Chapter 4, your genes don't dictate your health. You have the power to overcome them. You can make strategic lifestyle choices, such as the foods you eat or the supplements you take, based on your genetics, to optimize your health. You control your outcome!

It's pretty amazing what you can learn when you understand your genetic template. It helps guide your daily decisions. It becomes your blueprint to better health. It allows you to take a precision approach.

Back to my wealthy client, Eric. He didn't believe me when I told him that the food he was eating every day was killing him. But it was, and chances are what you're eating is killing you too.

Fortunately, Eric's desperation overcame his skepticism and he was willing to try just about anything. I got him on a personalized nutrition plan, based on his unique genetic profile, that he could stick with.

And stick with it he did! Over the next year, Eric lost over thirty pounds. He regained his energy and sense of vitality. His testosterone got back into a normal range, and his erectile dysfunction was no longer an issue. The best part? Eric got these results without a single medication.

"But what if I don't know my genetics yet?"

No worries! It's time for some general, science-based nutritional strategies you can apply to your everyday life. As mentioned earlier, while there's no one-size-fits-all perfect diet, there are some basic guidelines that every man should follow. And if you apply them, regardless of whatever gene variants you may have, you'll see a marked improvement in your health and vitality.

So, how do you get there without going on some kind of crazy restrictive fad diet that leaves you "hangry" and agitated all day long? We'll start with the basics.

Let's focus on what you should be eating — real food. In simple terms, if it grew from the ground or had a mother, you can eat it. Better stated, eat whole foods that aren't processed and don't come in a package.

These foods are typically on the edges of your grocery store. These include foods such as fruits, vegetables, meats, fish, nuts, and beans. If it has any ingredients that you can't pronounce — especially preservatives or chemicals, it doesn't belong in your body.

Here are a few rules to go by:

- Limit, or avoid altogether, processed or refined sugar. It promotes inflammation, weight gain, diabetes and cardio-vascular disease, and is truly the biggest evil in our diet.

- Plant-based proteins should be the cornerstone of at least two of your three daily meals.

- If you choose to incorporate animal-based proteins in your diet:
  - They should be the condiment of your meal. Plants should be the main dish!
  - Focus on high-quality, organic products. You want pasture-raised or wild-caught animal products.
  - Focus on primarily lean meats and fish. Fish are great because they are filled with the healthy omega-3 fatty acids, and they have much less saturated fat than red meat.

- Limit dairy intake. I get that cheese and ice cream are delicious. But unless you're a calf, milk from a cow was not intended for your digestive system. And they're loaded with endocrine disruptors (more on this in Chapter 17). If you feel like you absolutely *need* some milk in your life, make sure it's organic and grass-fed. Better yet, try almond or cashew milk. It takes some getting used to, but your body will be so much better for it.

Now, let's talk about calories. We'll start with the old-school thinking that if you restrict your calories enough, you'll lose weight.

The problem with this theory is that all calories are not created equal. What do I mean by that? Well, for example, one hundred calories of broccoli is not the same as one hundred calories of macaroni and cheese. They don't affect your body the same way. Broccoli has nutrients that your body craves, while mac and cheese, though delicious, has little to offer in the way of nutrients.

The broccoli is also going to fill you up longer, whereas the macaroni and cheese will leave you feeling hungry again shortly after you've eaten it. Your stomach may be full, but your cells are still hungry because they have not been fed.

So, if you're thinking that we're not going to be counting calories, congrats, you guessed right. What are we going to do instead? We're going to focus on macronutrients and micro-nutrients.

CHAPTER ELEVEN

BUILDING BLOCKS (LIFESTYLE - NUTRITION)

L et's start with macronutrients, the building blocks of nutrition. If your body is that Ferrari engine that runs on fuel, then macronutrients are the fats, proteins, and carbohydrates that provide that fuel. Simply put, your body requires macronutrients just to survive.

Now, let's talk a bit about fats. You may remember the low-fat craze of the 1980s. That diet fad led to a significant increase in obesity, so we learned that fat isn't the demonic beast it was made out to be.

The '80s may be far behind us, but the concept that fat is evil still haunts some people, so much so that they avoid even good fats like the plague. It's time to put an end to that myth once and for all and understand that our body actually needs good, healthy fats. Notice I said "good fats." Yes, the kind of fat matters, and I'll explain shortly.

As I've said throughout the book, everything in our bodies is interconnected. For example, the process by which your body makes testosterone starts with cholesterol; therefore, without good fats, your body literally can't make testosterone.

Hopefully that got your attention!

Now, let's turn to the proper breakdown of macronutrients. In general, an ideal starting point is 50% carbs, 30% fat, and 20% protein. By this I mean 50% of your calories should come in the form of good complex carbs (not simple, refined carbs or sugar!),

30% of your calories should come in the form of healthy fats, and 20% of your calories should come in the form of healthy proteins.

It's important to point out that this will need to be adjusted based on your unique genetics as well as your individual goals, but it's a great starting point for any guy. Now let's talk a bit about each of the macronutrients, and the best way to get enough of them in your body every day.

You may be surprised that I am encouraging so little protein, given all the talk of how your body needs protein to build muscle. Well, remember Popeye? Notice that he always downed a handful of spinach, NOT a slab of beef. Granted, Popeye was a fictional cartoon character, but whoever invented him actually had the right idea.

Like fats, carbs have also been vilified; and like fats, this is because people lump them all into one category. Most think of carbs as crackers, donuts, pasta and candy-filled snacks, but those are a subset of carbs called simple or refined carbs and, yes, they should be avoided except as a rare treat.

The reason for this is that those are simple sugars, and your body breaks them down easily, causing your blood sugar and insulin levels to spike. And remember that insulin levels are closely related to obesity because it's insulin's job to turn carbs into stored fat instead of energy that your body can use right away.

What you want to eat instead are complex carbohydrates like vegetables, fruits, and whole grains. They're digested and metabolized slowly in your bloodstream, leading to a slower release of healthy sugars. They don't cause your insulin level to rise dramatically, so you can use them as energy rather than storing them as fat.

Some of the healthiest complex carbs to incorporate in your diet are:

- All veggies
- Black beans
- Legumes
- Quinoa
- Steel cut oats (oatmeal)
- Sweet potatoes
- Fresh fruit
- Dried fruit (with caution — there is often tons of added sugar!)

Vegetables have a really high water content, so they contain fewer carbs than fruits, but both are crucial to a healthy lifestyle, as they're both loaded with lots of fiber, micronutrients, and lots of natural vitamins that your body craves.

Remember that your genetics, such as the PLIN-1 gene, can help us refine exactly how much complex carbs should be incorporated into your diet to help you burn fat, build muscle, and reach your goals.

Now let's get back to fats, beginning with the three types — saturated, polyunsaturated, and monounsaturated.

Saturated fats are found mostly in meat, eggs, and dairy. These have the potential to raise LDL and total cholesterol, encourage weight gain, and put you at risk for type 2 diabetes and heart disease, so you definitely want to eat them in moderation. Less than 10% of your "fat" calories should come from saturated fats.

Polyunsaturated fats include omega-3 and omega-6 fatty acids. Omega-3 fatty acids fight inflammation, so you want to load up on those. Omega-6 fatty acids tend to do the opposite — they promote inflammation — so you want to limit those. Examples of good healthy omega-3 fatty acids are salmon, flax seeds, chia, almonds, walnuts. Examples of omega-6 fatty acids are corn oil and sunflower oil.

We can actually measure the levels of omega-3 and omega 6-fatty acids in your bloodstream and work on optimizing it toward a healthy balance. A goal should be to get your omega-6 to omega-3 ratio under 4:1.

Monounsaturated fats are the healthiest type of unsaturated fat. They tend to raise "good" cholesterol (HDL) and lower "bad" cholesterol (LDL). These fats are typically found in olive oil, nuts, seeds, and avocados.

Now, let's talk about one more kind of fats that you want to avoid: trans fats.

Trans fats are manufactured, man-made fats that are used to make processed and fried foods and, ideally, should be completely eliminated from your diet. They increase your total cholesterol, LDL, and triglyceride levels and promote obesity and chronic inflammation.

One way to tell if your food contains trans fats is seeing the word "hydrogenated" on the label. Think of that as a skull and crossbones, because it's poison to your body.

To recap, here are some good, healthy fats that you should be eating:

- Avocados
- Chia seeds
- Fatty fish (salmon, trout, mackerel, sardines, herring)
- Nuts (almonds, walnuts, cashews)
- Olive oil (extra virgin)

Avocados and olive oil are some of the healthiest fats you can consume. Avocados contain mostly monounsaturated fats as well as other good stuff, like folate, vitamin E, and protein. Extra virgin olive oil is another great source of fat to add into your diet. It's loaded with monounsaturated fats, antioxidants, and has huge anti-inflammatory properties. Just be sure to pick a dark bottle to protect the oil from oxidation in the sun.

Remember, your body absolutely needs fats in order to make testosterone, but it's important to maintain a proper balance of good, healthy fats. Too much saturated, polyunsaturated omega-6, or trans fats can lead to inflammation, weight gain, and decreased testosterone production.

Genetics play a huge role in determining your individual response to fats in your diet. For example, your APOA5 (Apolipo-protein A-V) gene indicates how well your body responds to polyunsaturated fats. Knowing your APOE gene status is critical to understand your risk of vascular disease and Alzheimer's Disease with intake of saturated fats.

Now, let's talk about protein. Protein holds the lowest percentage of your daily macro intake, but it's still crucial to get enough of it every day. It goes a long way towards helping you feel full after a meal, plus it helps build muscle, along with healthy skin, hair, and nails.

Eating too much protein can actually raise cortisol levels (your stress hormone) and lower testosterone levels. Bottom line, when it comes to protein you need to know when enough is enough and stay within those parameters.

So what, you may be asking, constitutes good natural sources?

The best forms of plant-based proteins include:

- Amaranth - Complete protein; high in manganese
- Black beans - High amounts of lysine and leucine
- Green peas - High in fiber, leucine, lysine, and glutamine

- Hemp seeds - Complete protein, high in GLA
- Lentils - Contains all 20 amino acids
- Nutritional yeast - Deactivated yeast, high in B12
- Pumpkin seeds - Complete protein; high in healthy fats, magnesium, lysine, and zinc
- Quinoa - Complete protein; superfood high in fiber, vitamins and minerals, and antioxidants
- Spirulina - Algae superfood

In case you're wondering (or groaning), no, I'm not insisting you go vegetarian or vegan. While the crux of your diet should be plant-based, it doesn't have to be limited to just plants.

The best forms of animal proteins include:

- Chicken breast, boneless and skinless
- Eggs, free-range and organic
- Halibut, skinless
- Salmon, wild-caught
- Steak, lean and grass-fed
- Tuna

Just like carbs and fats, there are numerous genes associated with your body's response to protein intake. Genes such as the FTO gene mentioned earlier and the LPIN1 (Lipin-1) gene indicate whether you will burn fat better with a high- or low-protein diet. That means with certain genetic profiles, it is not beneficial to eat large amounts of protein.

Remember, while the Male 2.0 Method includes some general guidelines to help you know what to eat, the key is a precise, personalized, data-driven approach. There is no perfect diet, but understanding your unique genetic profile will help us create the diet that's perfect for you!

CHAPTER TWELVE

THE LITTLE STUFF MATTERS (LIFESTYLE - NUTRITION)

N ow let's talk about micronutrients because macronutrients only tell half the story.

Micronutrients are essential elements, like vitamins, minerals, and antioxidants. Every system in your body — digestive, reproductive, nervous, immune, etc. — requires micronutrients in order to function properly.

Your body *needs* micronutrients just to stay healthy. Micronutrients play a role in:

- DNA synthesis and expression
- Metabolism and digestion
- Transformation of macronutrients into energy
- Bone mineralization and growth
- **Hormone production (including testosterone)**
- Cell rejuvenation
- Brain protection
- Muscle movement and repair

Getting the right daily dose of micronutrients reduces your susceptibility to disease. They are also critical for maintaining optimal hormone health, especially zinc, magnesium, selenium, and several B vitamins. In general, most men don't eat enough of these foods to get the needed supply of the micronutrients they need.

So where do we find these micronutrients? Surprise, surprise, they're found mostly in whole foods, like vegetables, fruits, and whole grains – as well as *sunlight*! I'll explain...

One micronutrient that deserves special attention is vitamin D, which is technically a hormone. Vitamin D is particularly important in bone, muscle and vascular health, and is critical to normal sexual function. Healthy vitamin D levels can actually "switch on" over nine hundred important genes!

Vitamin D is produced by your body when your skin is exposed to sunlight. Yet the biggest reason for vitamin D deficiency in men is a lack of sun exposure. It's also important to have adequate amounts of magnesium and zinc to convert vitamin D into the active form we need.

I have found that most men are deficient in several key micronutrients, which is why I generally recommend good vitamin supplementation. Here's where epigenetics once again comes into play. There are genes related to your body's absorption and metabolism of micronutrients, and your unique genetic blueprint helps guide that decision.

For example, the FUT2 (Fucosyltransferase 2) gene controls your body's absorption of Vitamin B12. The cytochrome P450 gene, CYP27B1, is responsible for conversion of vitamin D precursors into the active form, whereas the VDR fok (vitamin D receptor) gene is important for vitamin D to activate its receptor and have a cellular effect.

The GSTP1 gene, for example, suggests increased risk of inflammation with Vitamin E supplementation. So as you can see, your unique genetic blueprint has a significant effect on your micro-nutrient needs and response to supplementation.

Remember to check out that FREE Male 2.0 Guide at drtracygapin.com/book for a cheat sheet and specific tools to help you optimize your nutrition, as well as how you can get your genetic blueprint done.

Now that we've gone through what to eat, what not to eat, and what proportions to eat it in, let's move on to an equally important factor in your nutrition: *when* to eat.

CHAPTER THIRTEEN

TIMING IS EVERYTHING (LIFESTYLE - NUTRITION)

You probably remember the old school thinking that we should eat five or six tiny meals throughout the day, presumably to keep our bodies from storing any excess food as fat. You may have even adopted this practice.

We now understand, however, that grazing all day is not optimal. As you will see, the key to optimal health is actually in time-restricted feeding, otherwise known as fasting. When you fast, you give your body an opportunity to use all the nutrients you've put into it, while also giving your digestive system a break.

You may immediately associate fasting with hunger pangs, light-headedness, and low energy. But I'm not talking about fasting for days and putting yourself into starvation mode.

I'm talking about *intermittent fasting*, which is a schedule with defined times for eating and the remaining time for digestive rest. Intermittent fasting is fairly easy to incorporate into your daily routine, and a major game-changer in anyone's health journey.

Digestion is a very energy-intensive process. If you're constantly eating, your body is putting energy towards digestion that you could use in better ways — building muscle, burning fat, making hormones, etc.

I want to stress that intermittent fasting is not a "diet," something you do only until you reach your goal weight, but a way of life. It's about living with intention and keeping your ultimate goals — your WHY — in mind.

Unlike calorie restriction, intermittent fasting doesn't slow down your body's metabolism. Instead, it increases it and helps you burn even more calories. You burn fat while maintaining lean muscle mass. So, whether you're trying to lose one hundred pounds or just that last stubborn ten, intermittent fasting will put your body into fat-burning mode naturally.

Intermittent fasting has been shown to:

- Balance hormone levels
- Raise norepinephrine and epinephrine levels, which encourage fat breakdown
- Increase growth hormone levels, which grows and preserves muscle mass
- Strengthen skeletal muscle mass
- Lower blood glucose levels
- Decrease insulin levels and increase insulin sensitivity
- Increase lipolysis (breakdown of fats) and fat oxidation
- Enhance glucagon levels, which encourages breakdown of fat

Intermittent fasting has also been shown to expand both your healthspan and your lifespan. Intermittent fasting activates both the SIRT-1 gene and the AMPK gene, genes that are each considered the holy grail of health and longevity. It turns on the FOXO gene, another longevity gene that also increases levels of adiponectin, ultimately leading to reduced visceral fat.

Recent studies have shown that a key aspect of intermittent fasting is the need for adequate NAD+ levels to experience the full benefit. As I mentioned in Chapter 8, diminishing levels of NAD+ is a major culprit in the aging process. We now know that maintaining healthy NAD+ levels is also critical to experience the beneficial effects of intermittent fasting.

Intermittent fasting has been shown to turn off genes related to inflammation. There have also been several studies showing that it has a positive effect on testosterone levels.

So you see, there are a number of benefits to intermittent fasting, including reduced inflammation, improved hormone levels, fat loss, and the activation of a bunch of genes that expand your lifespan. And it has no downside, other than having to adjust to a more specific timeframe for eating throughout the day.

This topic brings to mind a former patient named Ron, who had come to me for erectile dysfunction. Ron was carrying quite a bit of extra weight, but he didn't seem to be able to do anything about it. He insisted that he exercised and ate well, but he just couldn't get the weight off.

I suggested Ron try intermittent fasting. He didn't have to change anything he ate, he merely had to change the time that he ate it. Ron noticed weight loss almost immediately. He was blown away that simply changing his eating schedule could have such a profound effect on his health.

I wasn't surprised. The truth is that we're always in one of two states — fed or fasted. When we're in a fed state, our insulin levels are elevated. And when our insulin levels are elevated, our body tends to store fat rather than burn it.

When we're in a fasted state, however, our insulin levels drop, allowing our body to tap into its fat stores as a source of energy. This helps increase your energy, improve metabolism, and burn fat.

So, how do you incorporate intermittent fasting into your life?

There are several methods of intermittent fasting, including:

- **Skipped meals**: skipping one meal, typically breakfast. This is the easiest way to start intermittent fasting.

- **Eating windows**: condensed food intake to 8 hours (or less if you can!) for the entire day, while the rest of the day is fasting. This is termed "16:8 intermittent fasting" — fast for 16 hours and eat for 8 hours.
- **Warrior fast**: condensed eating window to 4 hours or less, preferably early in the day to allow your gut time to rest before sleeping
- **24/48 fast**: avoid eating for a full day or two — I recommend this at least once a month.
- **5-2 fast**: eat regularly for five days and then less than 600 calories for 2 days per week (can be consecutive or spread throughout the week).
- **Alternating fast**: eating regularly for 24 hours and fasting for 24 hours in rotation

What I typically recommend to clients and patients is the 16:8 fasting schedule, because it's the easiest to follow and requires the least amount of adjustment when you get started.

Most men skip breakfast, break the fast with lunch, and then enjoy dinner. Then you'll fast for the next sixteen hours, which is just enough to put your body into autophagy. Remember autophagy from Chapter 8? It's that process where your body clears away dead cellular debris so your healthy cells can function properly.

I want to stress that this practice does not require you to reduce your calorie intake during the feeding window, though most people find that they tend to eat less.

So, what might your day look like when you're living on an intermittent fasting schedule?

- Skip breakfast. You can drink black coffee, herbal tea and water. No sugar or creamer in your coffee, but plant-based stevia is okay.
- Break your fast around eleven a.m. or noon.

- Consume all of your daily calories, macros and micros during your eight-hour feeding window. This typically includes lunch and dinner. Begin your fasting window no more than eight hours after you broke your morning fast.

If you can't quite commit to this on a daily basis, start by doing it one day a week and then every other day. It won't take long for you to see the benefits, and that should convince you to make intermittent fasting a daily practice.

Remember how I told you that intermittent fasting will turn your body into a fat-burning machine? Well, there's even more you can do to get the most out of your nutrition plan. You can take it up a few notches by adding in carb cycling.

I've included your intermittent fasting checklist in the Male 2.0 Guide that goes along with this book — you can download it for FREE at drtracygapin.com/book.

Carb Cycling

As its name suggests, carb cycling is changing up how much carbs you eat on a daily basis. It includes specifically planning your carb intake around your workouts — more on this in Chapter 16.

Let's talk about what your body does with carbohydrates. Carbs are fuel that your body uses for energy. But what happens to excess carbs that your body doesn't turn into energy? Yep, you guessed it — they get stored as fat (along with glycogen) to be used at a later time, when your body needs more energy.

If you're constantly giving your body a steady supply of carbs, it will never need to break down that stored fat. This is why carb cycling is so beneficial — it mimics the body's natural cycle by encouraging it to break down its fat stores.

On your "low carb" days, you're depleting your body's glycolgen stores. Since you're not adding any more carbohydrates to your body, it has to tap into fat reserves to get fuel. You can amplify this effect by exercising on these days, so you're really depleting your body's glycogen stores and burning fat.

On "high carb" days, you have higher carbohydrate intake (complex carbs of course!), and your body gets the nutrients it needs to rebuild your energy stores. Here's the thing — for energy, your body consumes glycogen first and then fat, so it will replace glycogen *before* storing fat. When you combine carb cycling with intermittent fasting, your body becomes incredibly efficient at burning fat.

Carb cycling also provides additional benefits, including:

- Increasing your metabolism
- Lowering your body's insulin levels
- Helping counteract insulin resistance
- Training your body to burn excess carbs, not store them as fat
- Enhancing energy levels

Now let's talk about how to do this...

- On low carb days, you'll consume **50 net grams of carbs or less** and do high intensity interval or speed-burst workouts.
- On recovery days and strength training days, you'll eat **a normal amount** of carbohydrates.
- On leg day, when we work the biggest muscle groups in the body (and burn a ton of calories), you'll eat **slightly more carbohydrates**.

When you cycle through these three carbohydrate levels you turn your body into a fat-burning furnace. We'll talk a lot more about the exercise component in Chapter 16, but here's an example of what it looks like:

- *Monday*: low carb, high intensity interval training
- *Tuesday*: low carb, sprints
- *Wednesday*: normal carbs, strength training
- *Thursday*: normal carbs, strength training
- *Friday*: normal carbs, rest or active recovery
- *Saturday*: high carb, leg day!
- *Sunday*: normal carbs, rest or active recovery

So you can see how the Male 2.0 Method focuses not only on eating the right foods, but also on eating at the right times and pairing it with your exercise routine – all of which are powerful tools to burn fat, build lean muscle, and optimize your health.

Now let's dive into something that we all live with and many men find difficult to talk about — stress.

CHAPTER FOURTEEN

UNDER ATTACK
(LIFESTYLE - STRESS)

"I've suffered a great many catastrophes in my life. Most of which never happened."

–Mark Twain

I recall a time not too long ago when I took my two young children jet skiing on a big lake in Georgia. They were both having an absolute blast, squealing with delight as we coasted through the water.

But I wasn't enjoying myself quite as much. All I kept thinking about was all the patients with injuries from jet ski accidents I'd treated during my surgical career.

I was breathing fast, my heart was racing, and my jaw was clenched. I had this odd feeling of danger all around me, even though absolutely nothing was wrong. These are classic signs of stress, and I'm sure you've felt them before, even if you've never ridden a jet ski with two eager, fearless kids.

In today's world, men are stressed at unprecedented and extra-ordinary levels, often without them even being aware. We are expected to work crazy long hours, and whoever sleeps the least seems to have bragging rights. The hustle of hunting woolly mammoth to bring home for family dinner has somehow evolved into the hustle of an eighty-hour work week, with little focus on the importance of relaxation. And, as the Mark Twain quote above suggests, we're constantly worried about the future – stuff that hasn't happened and likely never will.

The problem with this (outside the obvious — that life is meant to be enjoyed) is that it leads to a state of chronic stress, and it's slowly but surely killing us.

What happens when we're stressed?

To simplify things, we humans have a sympathetic and parasympathetic nervous system, both of which work involuntarily, without our thinking about or realizing it. The sympathetic nervous system is responsible for that "fight or flight" feeling, like the caveman being chased by a tiger or a modern man worrying that his children are in immediate danger.

Your parasympathetic nervous system is responsible for what's called "rest and digest." It kicks in when you're at peace, meditating, or simply relaxed and promotes optimal health and balanced hormone levels.

These systems work together in harmony and counter each other. Each system is critical for your health at the appropriate times and situations, but in general, you want the parasympathetic nervous system to dominate.

When we're stressed, the sympathetic nervous system takes over. Adrenaline and other stimulating neurotransmitters get released. Heart rate, blood pressure and respiration all increase. Cortisol levels go through the roof.

As we discussed in Chapter 9, there's a big difference between acute and chronic stress. In the short term, acute stress is a normal, necessary response to an emergency situation. But the physiologic response to chronic stress promotes elevated glucocorticoid levels (specifically the stress hormone cortisol) and becomes harmful.

Chronic stress has been linked to:

- Inflammation
- Hormone imbalance
- Erectile dysfunction
- Hypertension/high blood pressure
- Cardiovascular disease
- Cancer
- Obesity
- Immune dysfunction
- Accelerated aging and early mortality

Chronic stress disrupts sleep and promotes high blood pressure. It leads to weight gain and loss of muscle mass. It affects our brain by altering function and connectivity.

Numerous studies have shown that chronically elevated cortisol from stress is directly linked to low testosterone. It not only inhibits testosterone production, but also raises SHBG (sex hormone-binding globulin), that protein we talked about earlier that reduces the amount of bioavailable free testosterone.

Chronic stress also crushes your ability to have normal erectile function through its effects on not just testosterone but also on neurotransmitter production and vascular function.

Research has shown that chronic stress affects us at an epigenetic level, by directly altering gene expression. It works through those processes I mentioned earlier, such as methylation or acetylation, that result in activation or deactivation of critical genes. It also increases the production of complex proteins such as NF-kB (nuclear factor kappa B). This leads to increased expression of pro-inflammatory genes, promoting chronic inflammation. This is how stress directly promotes illness and cellular aging.

Chronic stress has been found to shorten your telomeres, and therefore your lifespan! This means you're not only subjecting yourself to a constant feeling of being under attack, you're also ruining your health and your quality of life in the process.

Now that you understand some of the science showing the connection between psychologic stress, gene expression, disease risk, and longevity, let's talk about what you can do about it.

First, it's important to clarify exactly what we mean by stress. There is a stressful event — for example, missing your flight, getting a flat tire, or waking up late — and then there is the stress response, or your internal physiologic response to your environment. This is what we're talking about here, and the key to managing it is stress resilience, which is one of the key tenets of the Male 2.0 Method.

We all experience the kinds of stressful events mentioned above; life is far from simple and every day poses new challenges. It's how we frame stress in a proper perspective that counts. We cannot simply avoid stressful events; nor can we necessarily reduce the stress in our lives. To just ignore stress or pretend it doesn't exist is a basic feature of Male 1.0.

There was a recent study that asked a group of people how much stress they had in their lives and their perception of how that stress affected their health. What the researchers found was fascinating.

Those who believed that the stress in their lives affected their health died earlier than those who did not think their stress was harmful. This was the case even with those with high stress. It was not the actual number of stressful situations in their lives, but their *perception* of that stress, that affected their mortality.[3]

To be healthier, we don't need to get rid of stressful situations — that's not really possible anyway. Instead, we need to increase our stress resilience. This means learning how to embrace stress and to view it as helpful, not harmful.

The Male 2.0 Method views stressful events as helpful — as having a POSITIVE impact in your life, ones that can help you rise to the challenge. When viewed as useful, stressful events help you become stronger, more focused, and more intentional.

So how do we do this? How do we frame stress in a healthy perspective?

We activate your parasympathetic nervous system. Let's see how...

Meditation

One of the easiest and most effective ways to change our stress response is through relaxation practices such as meditation. Meditation has been shown to reduce cortisol and increase testosterone by altering gene expression.

Meditation relieves our subjective feelings of anxiety and depression and improves our mental focus and sense of well-being.

It's also been found that long-term meditation increases grey matter volume of the brain and enhances connectivity between brain regions, which translates into better cognitive performance.[4]

One study looked at the methylation pattern, an indication of epigenetic effect, of meditation. They found that long-term meditators had over 2200 genes that were positively affected by meditation. Even the novice group, who just went through eight weeks of meditation training, had over 1500 genes affected.[5]

Another recent study from Coventry University in England showed that meditation consistently reduced nF-KB levels, that marker of inflammation we talked about.[6]

As you can see, meditation has been proven capable of reversing the effects of chronic stress down to a genetic level. The brain is malleable, and meditation actually changes its structure by promoting neuroplasticity, the complex process by which the brain reorganizes through the formation of new neural connections.

Once I've explained all this to my patients, the first question they have is, "How do I meditate?" It's actually pretty simple! You relax, focus on your breath, and simply be present in the moment.

- Go to a quiet place where you won't be disturbed, sit comfortably, close your eyes, and just breathe.

- Focus on your breath. Breathe slowly with your belly, not your chest. We'll talk more about this in a moment.
- If you find your mind wandering, come back to the breath. Stay with the feeling of *the breath*.
- If something is going on in the world around you, take notice of it and then come back. Acknowledge the chirping birds. Smell the bacon cooking downstairs? Wait, bacon?! No, no. Come back and focus on the breath.
- You don't need to *stop* your thoughts...just guide them back to focus again on your breathing.

I recommend you try meditation once a day, five minutes a day, for thirty days. I promise you will have a clearer mind, with less stress and a better outlook on life. It will help you reconnect to what's happening around you and will radiate into every facet of your life from your work, to relationships, to exercise, to hobbies, and beyond!

Now, I understand that your job is demanding and your schedule nonstop. But ask yourself, what is the point of all this hard work if you can't even get five minutes to yourself to regroup?

You can meditate anywhere — at home, at work, or even in your car. There are even several apps for it!

Here are a few I recommend:

Headspace: This is a collection of science-based meditations, animations, articles, and videos to help you train your mind. This is the one I use, and definitely worth looking into.

Insight Timer: This app has one of the largest databases with over 13,000 guided meditations on topics like stress, relationships, creativity, productivity, and more. It also includes podcasts for inspiration and music tracks to soothe your mind. It's great for both short, stress-blasting bursts and long meditative sessions.

Calm: Tranquil sounds and music instantly relax you when you open the app. It offers shorter meditations, particularly those to help you sleep.

There are literally countless ways to meditate, so in addition to these you might do a little research on your own. Whatever method you choose, it will help reduce stress and mental chatter and retrain your brain to think critically, creatively, and clearly. You will be training your brain to let go of stressful thoughts and accept positive ones.

On my way home from work every day, I stop in a parking lot not far from my house. I park, close my eyes, and do ten minutes of meditation with my Headspace app. Then I'm able to go home to my wife and kids and be calmed, focused, and present for them. Just five to ten minutes has a huge effect — try it!

Breathing

Let's talk a little bit about breathing. Whether we realize it or not, nearly all of us are doing it wrong. Right now you might be thinking, "This is ridiculous, I know how to breathe!" Sure, you're breathing enough to keep you alive, but when we're talking about optimal health, there's actually a right way and a wrong way to breathe.

Most men breathe through their mouth instead of their nose; they use their chest and they breathe way too quickly. This is called over-breathing, and it can have a massive effect on your cognitive and physical performance. It leads to chronically depleted CO_2 levels, called hypocapnia. Nearly every client I work with has issues with over-breathing.

The CO_2 level in your bloodstream is critically important because it directly regulates the size of your airways, blood flow through your body (through dilation or constriction of your blood vessels), and the actual release of oxygen to your cells. So hypocapnia directly reduces tissue oxygenation through these mechanisms, and ultimately impacts your performance — both physically and mentally.

Here are some tips on how to breathe properly:

- You should always breathe in through your nose and out through your nose — never your mouth.
- Focus on belly breathing, not chest breathing. This means that your belly should go out as you inhale and come back in as you exhale. Your chest wall should never move when you're breathing. Chest breathing is actually really shallow breathing, whereas belly breathing enables more efficient gas exchange.
- When you exhale, you should almost have the sense that air is falling out of your body, rather than you pushing it out.

Let's look at a few breathing techniques that you can incorporate into your daily life as well as your meditation.

First is box breathing. You start by inhaling for four seconds (through your nose, of course). Hold your breath for four seconds, then exhale for four seconds. Then hold it again for four seconds and start over. Do this on repeat, and you'll feel a lot less stressed.

Another great breathing technique is to breathe in for four seconds, hold your breath for seven seconds, and then exhale for eight seconds. The purpose here is to train yourself to slow down your breathing and make you mindful about not over-breathing.

It may seem silly that I'm making such a big point about breathing because it's something that we don't normally think about. But increasing your CO_2 levels by focusing on proper breathing provides so many benefits, including increased heart rate variability (more on this soon!), improved cognitive clarity and focus, and most importantly, better stress resilience.

Exercise

Exercise has an amazing impact on chronic stress and cortisol levels. Working out also releases endorphins, which makes you happier and less stressed. Yoga is a great form of exercise because it focuses on proper breathing and promotes relaxation. A lot more on exercise in Chapter 16!

Spending time outside is also helpful for promoting a healthy stress response. Fresh air helps calm the mind and body. Studies show that walking in nature is linked to lower cortisol levels. In fact, many doctors in other countries actually "prescribe" nature as a way of improving health!

Sex

Another great way to reduce chronic stress is sex. Having sex releases endorphins and serotonin, which make you happier, less anxious, and more energized. It also helps reduce chronically elevated cortisol levels.

Sex helps burn calories and increase oxygenation, which could help you shed a few extra pounds, and sex before bedtime can help you have a more restful sleep. So your homework tonight is more sex!

Beyond that, go out and do things that you enjoy. Remember your WHY. Are you focused on it? If it's your children, for example, are you dedicating time to be with them?

This is a principle of the Male 2.0 Method that I keep coming back to — *living with intention*. What's it all for if you're not taking time to enjoy life? Schedule it, plan it, do what you have to do — just make it a priority.

For a cheat sheet on mastering stress resilience, check out drtracygapin.com/book and download the FREE Male 2.0 Guide.

One more incredible way to reduce cortisol levels and over-come the effect of chronic stress? Sleep!

CHAPTER FIFTEEN

DREAM ON
(LIFESTYLE - SLEEP)

We're living in an era where it's considered manly to get by on as little sleep as possible. We're encouraged to stay up late to get more work done, then get up extra early to get to the gym before work. To "hustle." And we're expected to be wide awake, powered up like the Energizer Bunny through all of it. The problem is that we're not battery operated, so it's really not working for us.

I get it because I used to be the same way. I'd be up till one a.m., getting some of my best work done, and I thought I was doing the right thing because I was super-productive at night. Then I'd have to drag myself out of bed early in the morning to get to the operating room.

I thought I was used to it, since I got by on very little sleep back in my residency days. But the truth was that I was miserable every day, struggling against exhaustion, relying on coffee just to get by, and I refused to even admit it to myself because that wouldn't be manly, would it?

Now, I make it a point to get to bed by ten-thirty p.m. because I require a certain amount of sleep. And so do you! And it has to be good quality sleep, too.

What happens when you don't get enough sleep? For starters, your metabolism slows down. Your body goes into survival mode, which means you store nutrients as fat and you can't build muscle.

The process of autophagy that we talked about earlier slows

down, so none of the senescent cells in your body are being cleaned out. Your body basically becomes a hoarder of half-dead, degenerate cells that pile up and wreak havoc on all of your systems.

Poor sleep has been found to be associated with reduced testosterone levels by as much as 50%.[7] Sleep deprivation also increases your risk of obesity, diabetes and chronic inflammation, and is strongly associated with Alzheimer's disease, high blood pressure, and a whole host of other illnesses.

Did you know that the World Health Organization (WHO) has classified shift work, meaning working overnight, as a carcinogen? Yes, it's true, and it takes substantial data for them to make such a classification.

Sleep deprivation also decreases attention and mental clarity and is much to blame for one of the top ten causes of death in the US — car accidents.

On the other hand, consistently getting good quality sleep provides massive benefits. In fact, just one good night of sleep turns over 500 healthy genes.[8] Imagine the benefits of getting a good night's sleep on a consistent basis!

So how much sleep do we really need? Everyone requires seven to nine hours of sleep a night. We hear all the time that we need eight hours of sleep, but that's just an average.

Many guys claim that they do just fine on six hours of sleep or less. But this is simply not true. You may become used to being sleep deprived and unhealthy, but you're certainly not functioning at your full potential. More on this when we talk about tracking sleep with wearable tech in Chapter 18, but the takeaway here is that good sleep has a MASSIVE effect on your performance.

We're not just talking about the quantity of sleep, but also the quality, as both directly impact your body's performance at an epigenetic level. Your metabolism, blood sugar regulation, hormone production, and autophagy are all affected by your clock genes, which are closely regulated by your sleep.

So what constitutes a good night of sleep?

There are multiple stages of sleep, each of which is important for different reasons. The sleep cycle starts with REM (rapid eye movement) sleep, which is the lightest stage of sleep and when you tend to dream. You then gradually transition into the four stages of non-REM sleep — two light sleep stages and two deep sleep stages — over a ninety to one-hundred-twenty-minute period. That said, deep sleep, which is characterized by slow brain waves, tends to occur more in the first half of the night, while REM sleep, characterized by fast, irregular brain waves, tends to occur more in the second half of the night. Again, each phase of sleep is important for different restorative purposes. Deep sleep, for example, helps imprint memory and restore growth hormone levels.

The goal is to get four to five good sleep cycles over the course of a night. When your sleep is altered, you miss these key benefits. And when it's disrupted, you have to start all over again at the REM stage. This causes you to lose that critical deep sleep stage that's so important for your body to restore itself.

So why do you lay there tossing and turning in bed, unable to get to sleep? Or why do you wake up often throughout the night and then have a hard time falling back to sleep?

Given all the studies we've discussed throughout the book, it should come as no surprise that there's science behind our sleep patterns as well, or that it once again involves our genetics. Indeed, there is a significant genetic basis to the quality and quantity of your sleep, and this is good news, because once you know your genetics, you can improve your sleep!

There are genes that code for your circadian rhythm, such as your CLOCK genes and PERIOD genes. These indicate whether you are a "night owl" who does better going to bed late, or an "early bird" who does better going to bed early and waking up early.

Melatonin, which is produced in your pineal gland, is one of many hormones involved in regulating your sleep cycle. Melatonin shuts off your active brain and gets you to sleep.

There are a number of genes involved in melatonin production. One of these genes is called AANAT. People with a variant of that gene will have lower production of melatonin and consistently struggle to get to sleep.

Another gene related to inducing sleep is the ADA gene. In your brain, adenosine increases the activity of the AANAT gene. The ADA gene codes for enzymes that break down adenosine. Those who have a variant of the ADA gene don't break down adenosine as well, and actually have increased melatonin production and better sleep.

Have you ever wondered why drinking coffee has a way of waking you right up? Well, caffeine blocks adenosine at its receptor, therefore indirectly lowering melatonin levels. That disrupts the cycle and leaves you wide awake.

Men with a variant of the ADORA2A gene, which codes for the adenosine receptor, will be much more sensitive to caffeine than others.

We talked in Chapter 10 about the GAD-1 gene and how it can affect sleep. Remember that the GAD-1 gene codes for proteins that are involved in the breakdown of glutamate (an excitatory neurotransmitter) to GABA (a relaxing neurotransmitter).

People who have a variant of this gene tend to have a hard time falling asleep if they eat foods high in glutamate (i.e. wheat, grains, eggs, chicken, and any food high in protein) close to bedtime. Pasta (in small amounts!) may be fine earlier in the day, but if it's eaten at dinner they might find sleep eludes them that night.

The good news is that they will notice a *huge* improvement in their ability to fall asleep and stay asleep simply by altering their diet — specifically at night. Remember, when it comes to your genetic profile, knowledge is power!

That said, there are some things you can do to immediately improve your sleep even without knowing your genetic blueprint. A crucial aspect of this is what we call "sleep hygiene" — a set of daily habits to help you fall asleep fast and stay asleep.

Here are some general recommendations:

- Set a daily bedtime and wake-time schedule and stick to it. It should be the same during the week and weekend!
- Your bedroom should only be used for sleep and sex. Your mind will associate your actions with your environment. It's not a place to lie around watching tv or getting work done.
- Get your electronics out of your bedroom. Sleeping with them next to your bed disrupts your sleep through EMF energy, even if you don't realize it.
- The best sleep you'll get is in a completely dark room. Get some blackout shades, or a good sleep mask. Even clocks with lighting can be disruptive.
- Invest in high quality comfortable bedding — your sleep is worth it!
- Turn the A/C down — you'll get your best sleep when your room is extra cool.
- Practice the mindset or meditation techniques we've talked about before going to bed.
- Put away all electronic devices at least two hours before going to sleep. This includes your phone, laptop, and TV. The blue light disrupts melatonin production. You can also consider using blue-blocking glasses after sundown. Spend two hours before bed reading or meditating instead.
- Create a nightly ritual before sleep to turn off your analytical mind.
- Exercising and spending time in natural sunlight during the day will also improve your quality of sleep at night.
- Caffeine after two p.m. can destroy sleep quality — limit it as much as possible.

There are several supplements that have been shown to be helpful for sleep as well:

- Vitamin B6
- Magnesium Glycinate or Threonate
- Melatonin (although your genetics strongly influence your response)
- L-Theanine

These won't necessarily work for everyone, and are not intended as a replacement for good sleep hygiene, but they are certainly worth considering as an adjunct.

One more important point to emphasize here is that you need to be tracking your sleep — every single night. You want to know not just how long you sleep, but the quality of your sleep, which means tracking the stages of sleep described above.

There are numerous wearable devices that are great at tracking your sleep. I recommend the Oura ring or Garmin Fenix watch.

The Male 2.0 Method is all about using data to drive decisions. It's about personalization of your health. It's about being intentional about your health. And it's about leveraging epigenetics to optimize your health.

What helps other men sleep may not work for you. By tracking your sleep, you can relate it to your health and lifestyle choices and make changes in that work for you. We'll talk a lot more about tracking your sleep and other health data in Chapter 18.

Remember guys, good sleep is critical if you have any interest in reaching your full potential. Skimping on sleep doesn't make you a hero or a hustler — it just turns you into a zombie with low testosterone, high cortisol, and belly fat.

Be intentional about getting good sleep and watch how much better you'll start to feel every day. And be sure to download your FREE Male 2.0 Guide with your sleep hygiene cheat sheet at drtracygapin.com/book.

CHAPTER SIXTEEN

WORKING UP A SWEAT (LIFESTYLE - FITNESS)

"But, Doc, I'm too busy to exercise."
This is an excuse I hear all the time. I also hear, "I'm too out of shape," or "Too old." I do understand that you *are* busy, and that it's hard to get started when you're out of shape, and that it was easier when you were twenty-one. I also realize that going to the gym can be intimidating, especially when you're just getting started and perhaps not feeling your most confident.

But here's the thing — to live long, be strong, and remain healthy, you *absolutely* need to exercise. This is not optional. Consistent exercise is the key to optimized health and vitality.

Remember that study I talked about earlier, that found that regular exercise over the course of six months led to positive epigenetic changes in 7000 genes? That's about one-third of your genome! You can positively alter the expression of one-third of all of your genes just by doing regular exercise.

What kind of exercise should you be doing? Once again, it's helpful to know your unique genetic profile, as this plays a role in determining your response to exercise. Here's a great example:

It's known that a large number of Olympic sprinters, including Usain Bolt, come from a particular county in Jamaica. Researchers looked at genetics to gain insight into why. They found that most Jamaicans have a variant of the ACTN3 (alpha-actinin-3) gene, which codes for the development of fast twitch muscle fibers, which sprinters obviously need. But they found that the particular county where all the elite-level athletes come from has high levels of aluminum in the soil. And aluminum epigenetically upregulates (turns on) the ACTN3 genes in the first and second trimesters of pregnancy.

This fascinating study provides further evidence that your genetics *plus* your environment combine to produce an outcome. And that you can leverage your genetics to improve your training and optimize your overall performance.

For example, the AMPD1 (Adenosine monophosphate deaminase 1) gene codes for enzymes involved in processing ATP during exercise. Remember ATP is our main source of energy. And the PPARGC1A (peroxisome proliferator–activated receptor-γ coactivator-1 α) gene codes for proteins involved in mitochondrial biogenesis. Men with variants of these genes may have increased fatigue after workouts and may benefit from specific supplementation to help mitigate that effect.

Genes such as SOD2, IL6 and TNF are associated with levels of inflammation that develop from exercise. Men with variants of these genes have slower recovery and benefit from antioxidants post-exercise. But men with faster recovery should not use antioxidants or they lose the benefits of exercise. So you can see how knowing your genetics is critical!

Beyond your genetics, though, there are some general recommendations I suggest for every guy.

My first word of advice is that if you're not already exercising at least three times a week just get up off your couch and do something. Do something that you can commit to *at least* three times a week, and that alone will be a great start.

Yes, you need to be lifting weights and interval training to get the most benefits. If either or both of those seem daunting, start with *something,* even if it's just power walking around your neighborhood. *Just get moving* and work your way up from there.

On the days you're not exercising, you still need to stay active. Go for a walk with the family. Play ball with your kids. Walk up the stairs at work instead of taking the elevator. Move every day!

As you get older, your focus needs to shift from endurance exercises to more strength training and high-intensity interval training (HIIT). Strength training and HIIT are vital for men because they help maintain muscle mass and boost testosterone production.

Muscle loss, or sarcopenia, is a critical aspect of aging that's associated with early mortality. Maintaining healthy muscle is critical.

Core strength should also be a key focus for men as they age. Your core muscles provide stability, reduce risk of injury, and form the foundation of your strength.

It's also important to coordinate your workouts with your nutrition. As we talked about in Chapter 13, carb cycling is a great way to provide enough nutrients for your heavy workouts but still maintain a good macronutrient balance. On days when you are doing HIIT or cardio, your carb intake should be lower than on the days when you do strength training.

One thing you want to avoid is overtraining. In general, you don't want to perform strength training of the same muscles on consecutive days. Exercise is physiologic stress, meaning it tears down muscle to make it build up stronger, so training too hard can actually be detrimental. Be sure to give your muscles an opportunity to recover.

A great exercise on lighter workout days is yoga. If you've never done yoga, it may seem easy, but it's actually an amazing workout for strengthening your core muscles, teaching proper breathing techniques, and improving sleep.

The biggest thing of all is to find activities that you enjoy, because this will encourage you to stay active. Play tennis, jog, go biking, whatever it is you like to do. Just don't stop.

And don't tell me that you're too old! I have clients in their nineties who are still active on a daily basis. In fact, this is how they got to their nineties! I don't care how old you are, you have to stay active and exercise regularly.

When you combine regular workouts with the nutrition plan I gave you earlier in this book, you'll become limitless.

CHAPTER SEVENTEEN

DETERMINED DETOX (LIFESTYLE - ENVIRONMENT)

D id you know that you're on the pill? Yes, I am talking about THAT pill — the one your wife or girlfriend is taking so that the two of you don't breed an army of kids. How do I know you're on the pill? Simple — it's in the water you drink.

You know where else you're getting estrogen? In the plastic water bottle you're drinking from. In the plastic containers your food is stored in. In the food you're eating. In your personal care products like laundry detergent, soap, and deodorant.

Why is any of this important? *Because it's crushing your testosterone.* Testosterone levels in men are plummeting at a population level and it's become a crisis. A true epidemic.

There was a recent longitudinal study that looked at testosterone levels in men, the Baltimore Longitudinal Study of Aging. This study followed over 1700 men for over fifteen years. Over that time, they found a substantial population-level decline in testosterone levels.

The median total testosterone level dropped from 500 to just under 400. That's a 22% drop, which was 1.2% per year! Most importantly, *bioavailable T, or free T, dropped 459*[8]

The study found that not only were men losing testosterone as they aged, which was not unexpected, but that same-age men from later eras had substantially lower testosterone levels than men decades prior. This means that a fifty-year-old man today, for example, has a markedly lower testosterone level than a fifty-year-

97

old man fifteen years ago.

This is not just a problem in the U.S. A longitudinal study out of Finland followed men for thirty years and revealed a 37% drop in T levels, and a study from Denmark showed similar findings. [10,11]

Moreover, these studies controlled for health and lifestyle factors, such as obesity and diabetes, that are known to affect testosterone levels. The dramatic decrease in testosterone levels persisted even after correcting these factors. Clearly there is something else going on, and it's going on around the world.

That something is endocrine disruptors — chemicals and toxicants in our environment that interfere with your body's natural ability to make and regulate hormones, including testosterone. They have also been shown to cause several other negative effects, including obesity, cancer, diabetes, depression, and immune dysfunction.

Endocrine disruptors work through four different mechanisms:

- They can mimic normal hormones and trick our body into over-responding, like turning on a light switch that can never turn off.
- They can block natural hormones from binding to their receptors and functioning properly.
- They can interfere with the production, regulation or breakdown of hormones, or
- They can alter the hormone receptors so they don't produce their normal outcome.

Endocrine disruptors specifically reduce free and total testosterone levels by blocking production as well as altering the hormone's receptors so they don't function properly, thus resulting in a diminished response.

Endocrine disruptors are literally CRUSHING men's health.

There are hundreds of known endocrine disruptors. The EPA estimates over 3000 synthetic chemicals are produced in the US each year, and over 90% of them lack real data on their true health impact. There are likely hundreds more endocrine disruptors than currently estimated.

Endocrine disruptors - Where are they?

Unfortunately, they're everywhere, including:

- Our drinking water
- Pesticides/fungicides/herbicides that are sprayed on the food we eat
- Personal care products, such as fragrances, cosmetics, sunscreen, lotions, laundry detergent
- Household products, such as cleaning products, lawn-care products, waterproofing products, and teflon cookware
- Industrial products, such as flame retardants (on clothes and furniture), paint, adhesives, detergents, building materials, chemicals for cars, and rubber materials
- Plastics, such as toys, water bottles, food containers, and electronics
- Paper receipts
- Food coloring
- Pharmaceuticals...yep, the medicine you think is supposed to make you better!

Now that I've gotten your attention, let's dive a bit deeper. Back to the birth control pill I mentioned.

Over one hundred million women worldwide are on birth control. It gets excreted in their urine and gets recycled back into our water supply because our municipal water treatment plants do a very poor job at filtering estradiol.

Estradiol is a tough little molecule that's difficult to breakdown and has a prolonged effect — like the light switch analogy I mentioned where it turns on the receptor and it never gets turned off. This is a big problem because estradiol has been shown to not only lower free and total testosterone levels but also to cause infertility.

Another endocrine disruptor we're exposed to on a daily basis is atrazine. Atrazine is the second most commonly used herbicide on crops here in the US besides glyphosate. It's used most commonly on corn and other grain crops.

Studies have shown high levels of atrazine in lakes, especially across the Midwest and it's been found to be a major contaminant in our drinking water because our municipal water treatment centers don't effectively filter it.[12]

So what's the problem with atrazine? The problem is that studies show atrazine chemically castrates frogs, even in tiny doses. And in many cases, it turns male frogs into female frogs.

Let that sink in – atrazine causes male frogs to become female, who actually laid eggs and reproduced. If it can do that to a frog, what do you suppose it's doing to you?!

And it's important to note that in the studies, male frogs become female frogs exposed to 200ng/L of atrazine, which are very low doses. The studies that detected atrazine in our water supply found levels as high as 34,000 ng/L![13]

Now let's talk about plastic. It's cheap, it's convenient, and it's everywhere. But there are evils lurking in plastic, namely, BPA and phthalates.

BPA, or Bisphenol-A, is most commonly used to make plastic water bottles. Globally, we go through *a million water bottles per minute,* and most of them aren't recycled.

BPA is also used to make baby bottles, plastic cups, plates, utensils, food storage containers, and it's in the lining of metal cans. It leaches into our food and water, especially when it's warm. It's also in the coating of paper receipts, and you're absorbing it through your skin just by touching it.

Some people have gotten wise to the toxicity of BPA, so they look for the words "BPA-free" on their plastic or metal products. Unfortunately, most of those products have Bisphenol-S, which is no less harmful.

BPA has become so pervasive that nearly everyone is affected. One study found metabolites of BPA in the urine of 90% of the people tested.[14]

What's wrong with BPA? Several studies have shown a significant effect of BPA on testosterone production. An interesting study out of Paris looked at male human fetuses that were between six and eleven weeks gestational age and were about to be aborted.

They took Leydig cell tissue from the testes of these fetuses and cultured them in various concentrations of BPA. Within the first few days, they found a significant difference in testosterone production.[15] So we know there's a strong, direct effect of BPA exposure on our testosterone production.

Now let's move on to phthalates. This is where things get really ugly because phthalates are arguably the worst among endocrine disruptor with respect to its effect on men's health.

Phthalates are most commonly used as plasticizers that increase the flexibility and transparency of plastic. In other words, this is what makes a plastic bottle bendy and clear.

Phthalates are found in:

- Personal care products, such as shampoo, nail polish, soap, and hair spray
- Cosmetics and fragrances
- Shower curtains
- Plastic toys
- Vinyl flooring

- Detergents
- Cleaning products
- Food packaging
- Adhesives
- Paint
- Raincoats
- Plastic bags
- Garden hoses
- Building materials
- Children's toys
- And worst of all, our drinking water

One study found that 29% of our drinking water contains phthalates because again, our municipal water plants aren't filtering them out.[16]

Another study found metabolites of phthalates in the urine of 98% of the people tested.[17] This means that nearly all of us have significant levels of phthalates in our bodies from our environment.

Several studies have shown that there's a correlation between phthalate exposure and low testosterone, infertility, cancers, and reproductive abnormalities.[18,19] So think about the plastic you use in your everyday life, and the effect it's having on you.

Depending upon your age, you may recognize the name of the next endocrine disruptor: DDT. Back in 1972, this insecticide was banned in the US because it was found to cause cancer. It has since been banned in most parts of the world except Africa, where it's still used against mosquitoes to prevent malaria. But DDT residue is still present in the US, especially in Florida.

A study out of the University of Florida[20] looked at alligators in Lake Apopka, which is adjacent to a factory that had a major DDT spill in 1980. A group of grad students, who clearly drew the short straw, got the job of hand-capturing one hundred forty alligators, some from the contaminated Lake Apopka and others from the non-contaminated Lake Woodruff.

As if capturing the alligators wasn't rough enough, they had to then press on their cloacas (an opening for the digestive, reproductive, and urinary of certain vertebrate animals) to determine which ones were male. Then they measured the alligators' penis size and drew their blood to measure their testosterone levels. (Don't worry, no alligators were harmed in the conducting of this experiment.)

The findings were staggering. The alligators in the contaminated Lake Apopka had a 50% decrease in their testosterone levels, and a nearly 25% decrease in their penis size compared to those in the clean Lake Woodruff.

Think about it — the DDT spill was over thirty years ago, yet the alligators were still suffering from the effects of it. So, you can only imagine what havoc DDT may be wreaking on you.

Now, imagine I told you that there's something that will significantly lower testosterone level within one hour of drinking it. What would you think? Some poison stored in a bottle with a skull and crossbones on it? Nope, not even close. The culprit here is milk — the kind you buy off the shelf at the grocery store.

In a recent study, young boys were given milk, then their testosterone levels were checked. Within just one hour, there was a significant decline in their testosterone levels.[22] This is the stuff you were told "does a body good."

Milk is stored in plastic-lined boxes or plastic containers made of BPA and phthalate. But there's more to it than that. The cow has typically been pumped full of hormones to grow faster and bigger. Beyond that, the cows are being fed grains that are infested with a fungus called mycoestrogen, which is yet another endocrine disruptor. And those grains have been sprayed with nasty hormone-crushing herbicides and pesticides. So, every glass of milk is a toxic cocktail that's destroying your testosterone levels.

Finally, let's talk briefly about phytoestrogens, which include soy and tofu and flaxseed. This topic can get a bit heated among the plant-based community, but facts are facts!

Soy is the second most genetically modified crop after corn. And why is it genetically modified? To withstand the effects of glyphosate. The worst part is that we're not even eating the natural, raw organic soybean. It's just a highly processed version of soy with significantly increased phytoestrogen content.

To put things into perspective, let's consider an animal study that measured the effects of soy intake on testosterone levels. One group was fed a phytoestrogen-rich diet, while the other ate foods without any phytoestrogens. After five weeks, serum testosterone levels were tested among both groups.

Can you guess if there was a difference? The phytoestrogen-rich food diet produced a 50% decrease in testosterone levels. This was just five weeks of eating the sorts of foods that you probably eat all the time.[21]

And it's not just testosterone levels. We're also seeing a dramatic decrease in fertility in men from eating soy products.

As you can see, endocrine disruptors are everywhere, and the combined exposure to these toxicants has a dramatic effect on your testosterone, your fertility, and your life. Worse yet, these toxicants don't operate independently. They have a cumulative effect.

We eat them, we wear them, we wash our clothes in them, we cook in them, we store our food in them, and we lather ourselves in them. They're everywhere.

We are living in a soup of endocrine disruptors, and they're attacking our balls from every direction.

So, men, what do we do about this? Just take this feminization lying down? Absolutely not! We start by mitigating exposure. Here's a solid list of ways to minimize, if not avoid, exposure to endocrine disruptors in your daily life.

- First, you simply cannot drink from plastic water bottles. Just don't do it. Use an activated carbon water filter for your drinking water and you can store it in glass or stainless steel water bottles.
- Lose weight! Estrogenic endocrine disruptors are stored in your fat, so shedding the weight will help eliminate these toxicants.
- Eliminate highly processed foods and focus on eating organic fruits and vegetables.
- If you eat meat, eat only grass-fed organic meats and wild caught seafood like salmon. Make sure your meat cuts are wrapped in wax paper rather than stewing in plastic.
- Eat food with no plastic contact.
- Limit dairy, butter and cheese unless it's organic and grass-fed. Almond milk or cashew milk are certainly better alternatives to cow's milk.
- Don't eat processed soy or flaxseed products.
- Limit dietary grains, especially corn.
- Avoid all plastics, especially for storing or microwaving food.
- Avoid foods in metal cans.
- Avoid all lavender and any scented personal care products.
- Focus on quality cleaning products, laundry detergents, and dryer sheets. (I'll show you how!)
- Focus on quality personal care products including deodorant, shampoo, soap and sunscreen. (I'll show you how!)
- Plastics are killing us through our coffee K cups — avoid them and drink only fresh brewed coffee.
- Avoid plastic cups, plastic-lined mugs, and utensils, especially for hot drinks/coffee/food.

There are some great apps that can help you know which cleaning and personal care products are safe to use. A great one is the Healthy Living app by the Environmental Working Group. You can search for recommended products or you can actually scan the barcode of products to see the ingredients.

But we can go one step further. In addition to limiting exposure to endocrine disruptors, it's also important for you to be sure your body's detox systems are working at their best. When your body is functioning at its optimum level, your body can resist the effects of these environmental toxicants.

Like every other aspect of upgrading to Male 2.0, epigenetics and personalized genomics come into play here. This is where I say you have to know your genes, because your unique genetics dictate how your body responds to endocrine disruptor exposure.

You have genes such as glutathione peroxidase (GPX1) and catalase (CAT) that are involved in the efficiency of your detox systems to fight off toxicants. You also have genes, such as IL6, involved in the inflammatory response your body has to exposure to endocrine disruptors, which can sometimes be worse than the actual toxin itself.

Knowing your genetics is valuable because it helps identify and correct blind spots or weaknesses in your body's response to endocrine disruptors. This enables you to take a personalized approach to optimizing your body's protection.

For example, men with a CAT gene variant have a poor response to certain toxicants. These men would benefit from a higher fat diet and green tea which upregulate, or turn on, that pathway.

Men with an IL-6 variant may have a significant inflammatory response to endocrine disruptor exposure, beyond what is healthy. These men would benefit from DIM or indole-3-carbinol supplementation. So, knowing your genetics is a key step in optimizing your detox response to these toxicants.

Endocrine disruptors are everywhere, and they're destroying your health a little bit each day. It's time for you to take control.

You need to limit your exposure. And you need to know your genetics. Most of all, you need to be intentional and take control of your health and vitality. That's the whole point of Male 2.0.

> *Check out the FREE Male 2.0 Guide at <u>drtracygapin.com/book</u> for the endocrine disruptor cheat sheet that will help you eliminate the effects of endocrine disruptors on your health and vitality. I'll also share how you can get your genetic blueprint done so you can know how to optimize your body's defense against endocrine disruptors.*

CHAPTER EIGHTEEN

WEARABLE TECH

Now we get to the really fun stuff! You know the difference between men and boys? The price of their toys. And as you guys know, some toys are worth every penny.

Remember back in Chapter 5, I told you that Male 2.0 is data-driven, and that when you upgrade to Male 2.0 decisions about your health are based on real-life data with no more guessing.

Well, genetics are a big part of that. Your unique, personal genetic blueprint provides the foundation of your health. It's the data that never changes. It's your starting point.

That said, you also need a way to determine whether all of the changes you're making in your life are working. You're going to feel amazing, that's for sure. But you need objective data to prove that you're making progress. That's where wearable tech comes in.

If we can measure it, we can manage it.

Wearable tech allows you to track key biometric data. In simple terms, biometric tracking provides real-time actionable data about your health and physiology that you can use to make changes in your lifestyle.

Let's start with the basics — what kind of data can you track? For some time we've been able to track the number of steps we take each day and the amount of time we exercise. But thanks to incredible advancements in tech, we can now go well beyond that.

One important biometric marker is your resting heart rate, which is a direct indicator of overall health. You can track this over time and find that it correlates with your overall level of health and recovery. But let's take it a step further.

Perhaps an even more valuable data point is your HRV, or heart rate variability. HRV is the variation in your heart rate from one heart beat to the next. Let's say for example that you measure your heart rate and it's 80. The truth is, it's not really 80, because it changes by microseconds each and every beat. One beat may be 80.02, the next may be 79.99, and the next 80.01, and so on.

Though it may not seem like it, this is actually a huge deal. Heart rate variability is constantly changing based on your level of health, fitness, stress, and recovery.

We talked earlier about your sympathetic versus parasympathetic nervous system, and how your parasympathetic system is focused on "rest and digest" and your sympathetic system is focused on "fight or flight." Well these two systems are both pulling in opposite directions on your heart rate.

Your parasympathetic system slows your heart rate and promotes healthy variation. Think of it as dynamic flexibility of your cardiovascular system. This is HIGH heart rate variability. Your sympathetic system stimulates your heart rate and suppresses variation in your heart rate. This is LOW heart rate variability.

A high HRV signifies your system is rested, calm, loose, healthy, vibrant, and ready to go. This is good! It's associated with a healthy hormone balance, weight loss, and decreased inflammation.

On the other hand, a low HRV signifies that your system is overstressed, tired, unhealthy, and not at its peak. This is not good. It's associated with elevated cortisol, chronic inflammation, weight gain, and altered hormone balance.

Let me give you a few examples of how to apply this data to real life.

Imagine you have a bad night of sleep, or you go out for dinner and have a few drinks. You will probably see your heart rate variability go down. And again, low heart rate variability is a sign of an overstressed, unhealthy system.

Or imagine you work out really hard one day. The very next day, your heart rate variability plummets because your body needs time to rest and recover. Your body is in a state of stress as it's trying to heal. In that case, your body will not respond well to another workout. You should take the day off or maybe do some yoga or light cardio.

On days that your HRV is low, and you know it's not from an intense workout the previous day, you can ask yourself, "What did I do that put my body into such a stressed state?" You will normally be able to identify the trigger and make specific changes to your lifestyle.

One of my concierge clients noticed his HRV consistently dropped every Friday, even when he didn't have a hard workout on Thursday. We went through every detail of his lifestyle until we were finally able to figure out what was happening.

Every Thursday was date night with his wife and he always had a few glasses of wine. The alcohol was affecting his system to the point of drastically lowering his HRV! Sure enough, when he cut out the wine, his HRV stayed high.

This is an example of how we use data to drive decisions. I'm not saying he can't ever have a glass of wine. But now he understands how it affects his performance, which helps him prioritize what's important and make decisions accordingly.

When your heart rate variability is high, you can analyze what you did the day before that worked well for your system. Your HRV is truly a window into the heart and soul of your health. And it's constantly changing, so you can adapt your lifestyle based on your data. Just having this knowledge allows you to give your body exactly what it needs, without any guesswork.

There's a great device called HeartMath® that can actually help you improve your heart rate variability (HRV). The device connects with your phone or laptop and monitors your HRV in real-time with a finger or earlobe sensor. The program takes you through breathing exercises to entrain proper breathing techniques, and you see immediate improvement in your HRV. It's a great tool — one that I recommend my clients use at least a few times a week.

Now let's move on to how you can measure something else that's vitally important to our health — your sleep.

Remember in Chapter 15 I talked about the importance of getting enough good quality sleep. This means going through four or five cycles of the various stages of sleep, from REM to light sleep to deep sleep, and back again. It's important that you get enough REM sleep and deep sleep throughout the night to get the full restorative, restful effects.

You may think you're getting great sleep if you fall asleep easily and stay asleep throughout the night. But how can you know for sure? Unless you're tracking it, you don't.

That's why tracking your sleep is a critical part of the Male 2.0 Method. You need to rely on precise, real-life data to guide your daily lifestyle rather than just guessing what is right for your body.

You may find that you're not sleeping as long as you thought. You may find that you're not getting enough deep sleep or REM sleep. Or you may find you have disrupted sleep, and you're never fully completing your sleep cycle. Again, without tracking, you just don't know.

Once you obtain your sleep data, you can analyze it to understand how your lifestyle may be affecting your sleep. Let me share an example of how you can use your data to upgrade your sleep.

You may find that you're suddenly having very poor deep sleep or severely disrupted sleep. You take a deep dive into your lifestyle, make tweaks and adjustments, and learn that what you've been eating for dinner is affecting your sleep, like we've talked about in previous chapters. You can then make the right choices for your body and confirm the effects with real data.

There are also great tools to track your exercise, beyond just the number of steps you take. You can monitor the intensity of your workouts to be sure you're pushing yourself hard enough. If you don't stress your body out of your comfort zone, you're never going to improve and advance.

You can also track oxygen delivery to your muscles while you exercise. This can let you know whether you're exercising hard enough to reap the benefits, but not so hard that you're over-training and risking injury.

Finally, there are fun new wearable devices that show promise for improving your brain function. These devices work through a process called neurofeedback to improve your brain's ability to learn and adapt. This is the neuroplasticity I mentioned earlier when discussing the benefits of meditation. Indeed, these devices may help you meditate better, improve your memory or cognitive performance, or even perform better in sports.

And this is just the beginning. Technology is advancing so rapidly that it seems new biometric tracking devices come out every other day. We need to embrace these cutting-edge tools, not only because they are fun, but because the data they provide is invaluable. And we've moved beyond simply wanting to "know" and on to doing something about it.

The FREE Male 2.0 Guide that goes with this book includes a list of some of the key biometrics you can track regularly to optimize your health and performance. Again, you can find it at _drtracygapin.com/book_.

When you upgrade to Male 2.0, life is no longer about guessing or following the herd. It's about focusing on your personalized health data, including what it means and what you can do to improve it.

CHAPTER NINETEEN

GOODBYE PHARMACEUTICALS, HELLO PEPTIDES

Okay, guys, now for the cherry on top. Peptides. If you haven't heard about them yet, it's time to learn, especially if you're currently taking prescription drugs. Why? Because peptides can provide incredible benefits without the side effects of pharmaceuticals, and in fact they have the potential to replace pharmaceuticals within the next ten years.

Peptides are amazing molecules that work with your body to create a very specific outcome, from weight loss to injury recovery to gut health. But before I tell you more, let me make a disclaimer — peptides are *not* magic beans that do all the work while you sit around on your couch and eat like crap. They will, however, enhance all the things that you're doing right.

So what are peptides, exactly? Peptides are simply short chains of amino acids. They can have as few as two or as many as fifty amino acids in a chain. A chain of fifty to one hundred amino acids is called a polypeptide, and a chain with more than a hundred amino acids is called a protein. These amino acid chains function as signaling agents to achieve a specific outcome while limiting any potential negative side effects.

There are over fifty naturally occurring peptides, such as insulin and growth hormone, but over 7000 peptides have been synthetically created through amino acid sequencing. New, exciting peptides are being developed every day, and tons of clinical research trials are being published every month demonstrating their safety and efficacy.

Peptides have tons of functional benefits, and the great thing about them is that they're not made to suppress symptoms of diseases like pharmaceuticals. They improve, optimize, and enhance your health, as well as extend your life. Some of the functions of peptides include:

- Reducing Inflammation
- Muscle gain
- Weight loss
- Cognitive function, memory
- Gut health
- Exercise recovery
- Musculoskeletal / joint repair
- Hormone optimization
- Erectile function and sex drive

There are a number of peptides that I often recommend for my concierge clients, depending on their unique needs. Here are just a few examples:

BPC-157 is a great peptide for reducing inflammation, especially in the gut and joints. It can be given orally, subcutaneously, or injected directly into an area of inflammation such as a joint. There are numerous research studies on BPC-157 showing its amazing anti-inflammatory effect with little to no side effects.

CJC-1295 is a growth hormone-releasing peptide that's often paired with another peptide called Ipamorelin, a ghrelin receptor peptide. These peptides work together to boost your body's internal production of growth hormone, leading to better sleep, weight loss, muscle-building, enhanced exercise capacity and recovery, and improved cognitive function. These peptides are well-researched and tend to be much safer and more effective than giving growth hormone supplementation directly.

Melanotan-2 is an amazing peptide that improves erectile function and libido in men and also increases sexual desire and arousal in women. PT-141, or Bremalanotide, was developed from Melanotan-2, and is even more effective at stimulating erectile function, even for men who don't respond well to oral drugs like Viagra or Cialis. It can actually induce an erection within minutes!

So, why aren't peptides all the rage yet? The simple answer is money. When pharmaceutical companies create a drug, they spend a lot of money testing it, they patent it, and then they sell it for big bucks.

A peptide, on the other hand, can't be patented. This mean they're all generic, and anyone who knows how to make a specific amino acid sequence can sell them. So, for large companies in the pharmaceutical business, there's often no appeal.

If you do a search online right now, you'll find numerous websites selling peptides. That said, you should exercise caution when buying from these sites. Why? Because the sequencing of these amino acids must be absolutely meticulous. Lack of purity and poor quality control with no oversight or third-party testing has already become a problem. This means that when you order from these places you have no way of knowing what you're actually getting.

I recommend you obtain peptides only from a reputable compounding pharmacy with a doctor's prescription.

Simply put, get to know peptides because they're the way of the future. They're cutting-edge precision medicine tools that allow unique customization of your health. They're specific to your needs and provide amazing benefits with little risk. And they're an exciting part of the Male 2.0 Method!

The FREE Male 2.0 at <u>drtracygapin.com/book</u> includes a list of the best peptides currently available to optimize your health and performance. Check it out today!

CHAPTER TWENTY

PUTTING IT ALL TOGETHER

I have now given you the blueprint to upgrade to Male 2.0. It's not about just eating more vegetables and exercising more. And it's *definitely* not a one-size-fits-all health program. It's so much more.

Becoming Male 2.0 is a change in how you think and how you live. You are living with intention, with a laser focus on your big WHY that drives you every day to be the most amazing, optimized version of yourself.

Upgrading to Male 2.0 means you're empowered, with complete ownership of your health and your life. You're proactive about your health and no longer wait until you're sick to seek out medical guidance. You leverage your genetics and take a personalized, data-driven approach to optimizing your health and vitality.

As Male 2.0, you reclaim the vitality you had back in your prime. You're no longer just a man, but THE MAN! You feel amazing, with high energy, great sex drive, and confidence in how you look and feel.

As you transform into Male 2.0, you unleash your full human potential.

I hope you've come to understand that we are facing a true men's health epidemic, and only YOU can turn it around.

Low testosterone is crushing us.

Poor nutrition is crushing us.

Inactivity and lack of exercise are crushing us.

Micronutrient deficiency is crushing us.

Poor sleep and high stress are crushing us.

And endocrine disruptors are crushing us.

We owe it to ourselves to do better. To stop simply reacting to symptoms and disease. To stop thinking that taking care of our own health is selfish or a waste of time. And we have to protect our balls, because if we don't, no one else will.

I'm incredibly passionate about helping men like you optimize your health, vitality and longevity. I hope I've inspired you to lock arms with me, get empowered and take action.

I leave you now with a personal story that dramatically impacted my life and underscores my commitment to men's health.

My brother-in-law John was larger than life. He had a huge presence physically, but he also had a huge heart.

Everywhere he went, people loved him. And according to him, every stranger was a friend he just hadn't met yet.

John knew what was important in life, and of the many profound things he said, one of my favorites was, "Make today your best day, because you don't get today back."

One morning, at the age of forty-nine, John dropped dead from a heart attack. We later found out that he had been in poor health for a while, but from the outside you never would have known.

He had been trying to self-treat his symptoms of low testosterone by following advice he learned online and from his friends. He thought he was doing what was best for his health, but he was doing so without the data he needed. In reality, he had no idea what he was doing and was just guessing.

And the world lost a great man.

This is what I know to be true...

You absolutely have the power to take control of your health and how long you can live. But to do so, you have to live with intention, seek proper guidance, and take action.

You could choose to do nothing and stay on your current path. Or you could make a decision to step forward, upgrade to Male 2.0, and transform your health and your life.

Now is the time. Don't waste another day to get optimized.

Because you don't get today back.

To your health,

Doc Tracy

AFTERWORD

N ow that you are ready to take charge of your health and life in a whole new way and upgrade to Male 2.0, we are here to support you.

Go to <u>drtracygapin.com/book</u> to download the FREE Male 2.0 Guide that goes along with this book. It includes easy-to-use cheat sheets with specific tips and tools you can start using today. You'll learn how you can leverage your genetic blueprint to optimize your health and reverse aging.

You will also have the opportunity to reserve your personal Male 2.0 Performance Consult with me or my team. Start living your newly optimized Male 2.0 life filled with limitless energy and vitality!

ACKNOWLEDGMENTS

Writing a book is harder than I thought but more rewarding than I could have ever imagined. The experience has been both internally challenging and fulfilling. None of this would have been possible without my amazing wife, Sara. She supported me and stood by me every step of the way as I've developed my business, ideas, and this book. She even let me take over date nights with fun discussions on epigenetics, peptides, and longevity. Thank you, baby. You're my rock.

I'm eternally grateful to Daniel Stickler, MD for being my mentor in the world of precision medicine and epigenetics. I value your wisdom, knowledge and guidance. I value the visionary path you've shared to change the world of health and medicine. Thank you to my fellow colleagues in the Apeiron Academy, especially Melissa and the others in the mastermind.

Thank you to everyone on the Gapin Institute team who has joined me to pursue my vision. Again . . . and again . . . and again. Special thanks to Leann Spofford, the ever optimal, always smiling dreamer, who is always full of amazing ideas and insight. I'm forever indebted to Angela Giles and Tracey Thompson for their editorial help, keen insight, and ongoing support in bringing my messages to life. Thank you to Ash Ahern for my book cover design. And thank you to Shanda Trofe, who knows how to navi-gate the ins and outs of Amazon and the publishing world.

To my family, thank you for always believing in me and providing me never-ending love and support.

To men everywhere who aspire to be better husbands, fathers and leaders, thank you for the inspiration to help support your path to optimal health and well being. You truly are who I started this venture for.

The world is a better place because of those who have the "limitless" mindset. Thank you!

REFERENCES

1. Richardson S, Hirsch JS, Narasimhan M, et al. (2020) Presenting Characteristics, Comorbidities, and Outcomes Among 5700 Patients Hospitalized With COVID-19 in the New York City Area. JAMA. Published online April 22, 2020. doi:10.1001/jama.2020.6775.
2. Lancet. 2019 May 11; 393(10184): 1958-1972.
3. Keller A, Litzelman K, Wisk LE, et al. Does the perception that stress affects health matter? The association with health and mortality. Health Psychology: Official Journal of the Division of Health Psychology, American Psychological Association. 2012 Sep; 31(5): 677-684.
4. Luders E, Cherbuin N, Kurth F. Forever Young(er): potential age-defying effects of long-term meditation on gray matter atrophy. Front Psychol. 2015; 5: 1551. Published 2015 Jan 21.
5. Dusek JA, Otu HH, Wohlhueter AL, Bhasin M, Zerbini LF, Joseph MG, et al. (2008) Genomic Counter-Stress Changes Induced by the Relaxation Response. PLoS ONE 3(7): e2576.
6. Buric I, Farias M, Jong J, Mee C and Brazil IA (2017) What Is the Molecular Signature of Mind–Body Interventions? A Systematic Review of Gene Expression Changes Induced by Meditation and Related Practices. Front. Immunol. 8: 670.
7. R. Leproult, E. Van Cauter. Effect of 1 Week of Sleep Restriction on Testosterone Levels in Young Healthy Men. JAMA: The Journal of the American Medical Association, 2011; 305 (21): 2173.
8. Jonathan Cedernaes, Megan E. Osler, Sarah Voisin, Jan-Erik Broman, Heike Vogel, Suzanne L. Dickson, Juleen R. Zierath, Helgi B. Schiöth, Christian Benedict, Acute Sleep Loss Induces Tissue-Specific Epigenetic and Transcriptional Alterations to

Circadian Clock Genes in Men, The Journal of Clinical Endocrinology & Metabolism, Volume 100, Issue 9, 1 September 2015, Pages E1255–E1261.

9. Thomas G. Travison, Andre B. Araujo, Varant Kupelian, Amy B. O'Donnell, John B. McKinlay, The Relative Contributions of Aging, Health, and Lifestyle Factors to Serum Testosterone Decline in Men, The Journal of Clinical Endocrinology & Metabolism, Volume 92, Issue 2, 1 February 2007, Pages 549–555.

10. Perheentupa, Antti & Mäkinen, Juuso & Laatikainen, Tiina & Vierula, Matti & Skakkebaek, Niels & Andersson, Anna-Maria & Toppari, Jorma. (2012). A Cohort Effect on Serum Testosterone Levels in Finnish Men. European journal of endocrinology / European Federation of Endocrine Societies. 168.

11. Andersson, Anna-Maria & Jensen, Tina & Juul, Anders & Petersen, Jørgen & Jørgensen, Torben & Skakkebaek, Niels. (2008). Secular Decline in Male Testosterone and Sex Hormone Binding Globulin Serum Levels in Danish Population Surveys. The Journal of clinical endocrinology and metabolism. 92. 4696-705.

12. Kalkhoff, S. J., Lee, K. E., Porter, S. D., Terrio, P. J., and Thurman, E. M. (2003) Herbicides and herbicide degradation products in Upper Midwest agricultural streams during August base-flow conditions. J Environ Qual 32, 1025-1035.

13. "Smalling, K. L., Reeves, R., Muths, E., Vandever, M., Battaglin, W. A., Hladik, M. L., and Pierce, C. L. (2015) Pesticide concentrations in frog tissue and wetland habitats in a landscape dominated by agriculture. Sci Total Environ 502, 80-90.

14. Calafat AM, Ye XY, Wong LY, Reidy JA, Needham LL. 2008. Exposure of the U.S. population to bisphenol A and 4-tertiary-octylphenol: 2003–2004.Environ Health Perspect 116: 39-44.

15. N'Tumba-Byn T, Moison D, Lacroix M, Lecureuil C, Lesage L, et al. (2012) Differential Effects of Bisphenol A and

Diethylstilbestrol on Human, Rat and Mouse Fetal Leydig Cell Function. PLOS ONE 7(12): e51579.

16. Net, S., Sempere, R., Delmont, A., Paluselli, A., and Ouddane, B. (2015) Occurrence, fate, behavior and ecotoxicological state of phthalates in different environmental matrices. Environ Sci Technol 49, 4019-4035.

17. Zota, A. R., Phillips, C. A., and Mitro, S. D. (2016) Recent Fast Food Consumption and Bisphenol A and Phthalates Exposures among the U.S. Population in NHANES, 2003-2010. Environ Health Perspect.

18. Arbuckle, T. E., Fisher, M., MacPherson, S., Lang, C., Provencher, G., LeBlanc, A., Hauser, R., Feeley, M., Ayotte, P., Neisa, A., Ramsay, T., and Tawagi, G. (2016) Maternal and early life exposure to phthalates: The Plastics and Personal-care Products use in Pregnancy (P4) study. Sci Total Environ 551-552, 344-356.

19. Crinnion, W. J. (2010) Toxic effects of the easily avoidable phthalates and parabens. Altern Med Rev 15, 190-196.

20. Guillette LJ Jr, Parrott BB, Nilsson E, Haque MM, Skinner MK. Epigenetic programming alterations in alligators from environmentally contaminated lakes. Gen Comp Endocrinol. 2016; 238: 4–12. doi: 10.1016/j.ygcen.2016.04.012.

21. Maruyama, K., Oshima, T. and Ohyama, K. (2010) Exposure to exogenous estrogen through intake of commercial milk produced from pregnant cows. Pediatrics International, 52: 33-38.

22. Weber, KS., Setchell, KD., Stocco, DM., & Lephart, ED. (2001) Dietary soy-phytoestrogens decrease testosterone levels and prostate weight without altering LH, prostate 5alpha-reductase or testicular steroidogenic acute regulatory peptide levels in adult male Sprague-Dawley rats, Journal of Endocrinology, 170(3), 591-599.

ABOUT THE AUTHOR

Tracy Gapin, MD, FACS is a world renowned men's health & performance expert, professional speaker, entrepreneur and author. He has over 20 years of experience focused on providing Fortune 500 executives, business leaders, entrepreneurs, and athletes a personalized path to optimizing their health and performance.

Dr. Gapin incorporates precision hormone optimization, peptide therapy, state-of-the-art biometric tracking, epigenetic coaching, and cutting-edge age management protocols to help men not just optimize their testosterone levels but transform their health and vitality and reverse aging so they can be the most amazing version of themselves. As a renowned speaker, Dr. Gapin shares his signature talk: *Discover the Critical Drivers to High Performance in Every Area of Your Life.*

Dr. Gapin is board-certified by the American Board of Urology and is a Fellow of the American College of Surgeons. As a surgeon, Dr. Gapin pioneered a comprehensive program for advanced prostate cancer detection and treatment. He utilizes advanced biomarkers, multiparametric prostate MRI imaging and MRI-targeted fusion biopsy for prostate cancer detection and HIFU (High Intensity Focused Ultrasound) for prostate cancer treatment.

In 2017, Dr. Gapin created the Gapin Institute for High Performance Medicine to provide executives, entrepreneurs, business owners and athletes the data-driven solutions they need to optimize their bodies and brains for peak performance.

He also created individual and corporate health optimization programs, including his proprietary N1 Performance Health Program and the High Performance Health Conference.

Dr. Gapin is a member of the American Academy of Anti-Aging, Age Management Medical Group, The International Peptide Society, and the American Urological Association.

He lives in sunny Florida with his wife and two kids. He enjoys golf, tennis, skiing, and being the best father and husband possible.

To learn more about Dr. Gapin, please visit drtracygapin.com.

Connect with Dr. Tracy Gapin:

www.drtracygapin.com
www.gapininstitute.com
info@gapininstitute.com

Supplemental Guide to this book:

www.drtracygapin.com/book

LinkedIn: Tracy Gapin, MD

Twitter: @DrGapin

Facebook: @DrTracyGapin

YouTube: @DrTracyGapin

Instagram: @DrTracyGapin